Transdiagnostic Approaches in Cognitive Behavioral Therapy

Ana Claudia Ornelas
Editor

Transdiagnostic Approaches in Cognitive Behavioral Therapy

Springer

Editor
Ana Claudia Ornelas
Sunshine Therapy
Malden, MA, USA

ISBN 978-3-031-63493-2 ISBN 978-3-031-63494-9 (eBook)
https://doi.org/10.1007/978-3-031-63494-9

This Springer imprint is published by the registered company Springer Nature Switzerland AG
The registered company address is: Gewerbestrasse 11, 6330 Cham, Switzerland

Foreword

Cognitive behavioral therapy (CBT) has long been regarded as a cornerstone in the field of mental health treatment, offering effective interventions for a wide range of psychological disorders. Over the years, CBT has evolved, incorporating new approaches and techniques to address the complexities of human experience. In recent years, there has been a growing recognition of the importance of transdiagnostic approaches in mental health treatment. The emergence of transdiagnostic approaches within CBT, recognizes the common underlying mechanisms across different diagnostic categories and aims to provide tailored interventions that address core cognitive, emotional, and behavioral processes and transcend traditional diagnostic boundaries.

This book aims to provide a comprehensive overview of cognitive behavioral therapy (CBT) and its transdiagnostic approaches, offering a valuable resource for students and professionals working in the fields of psychology, mental health, and social work. The main idea is exploring the various transdiagnostic protocols and evidence-based interventions within the framework of CBT, emphasizing individualized treatments that focus not only on diagnostic labels but also on the unique characteristics and needs of each client.

Each chapter of this book delves into specific aspects of CBT and its applications, providing insights into the history of CBT, transdiagnostic approaches, case conceptualization, and various specialized interventions. The reader will find precious historical material about how, over the years, CBT has developed ways of dealing with uncomfortable emotions that could lead to loss of control. Several approaches are presented, in order to offer this clinical panorama towards a transdiagnostic intervention, like mindfulness-based cognitive therapy, dialectical behavior therapy, acceptance and commitment therapy, etc.

A special mention should be made to the conceptualization chapter, as it is a necessary condition for the application of any intervention protocol. Another strong point of this work, is that each chapter offers a deep dive into the theoretical foundations, methodology, and practical techniques of these interventions. In other words, in this book, we delve into the realm of transdiagnostic approaches in cognitive behavioral therapy, exploring how these approaches have revolutionized the way we conceptualize and treat psychological disorders. Through a series of comprehensive chapters, one can examine the theoretical foundations, clinical applications, and empirical evidence supporting transdiagnostic interventions in CBT.

One of the unique aspects of this book is its emphasis on the collaboration between therapist and client in developing a therapeutic alliance and working towards emotional regulation. Through case conceptualization and evidence-based interventions, therapists and clients can navigate through emotional distress, develop coping strategies, and achieve positive outcomes.

Furthermore, this book highlights the importance of integrating research findings and clinical expertise to inform evidence-based practice. In an overview you will find:

Chapter 1 takes us on a journey through the history of CBT, tracing its evolution from the traditional models of the 1970s to the emergence of contextual therapies in the 2000s. The authors explore the concept of emotional regulation achievement and its pivotal role in managing psychological distress.

Chapter 2 introduces us to transdiagnostic approaches within CBT, highlighting their multidimensional models and emphasis on shared mechanisms of diagnosis conditions and comorbidity disorders. The reader can explore how these approaches promote emotional regulation strategies and enhance clients' ability to modulate emotional experiences.

Chapter 3 delves into the importance of case conceptualization and therapeutic alliance in CBT, emphasizing their role in guiding treatment planning and fostering a collaborative relationship between therapist and client. The importance of this chapter lies in the fact that a tailored intervention depends on fundamentally of a precise case's comprehension.

Chapter 4 explores the contributions of functional analytic psychotherapy (FAP) to transdiagnostic interventions in CBT, focusing on the therapeutic relationship as a catalyst for interpersonal and intimacy repertoires.

Chapter 5 examines mindfulness-based cognitive therapy (MBCT) as a tool for managing experience avoidance, cognitive fusion, and rumination, offering insights into its applicability across a wide range of psychological disorders.

In Chap. 6, the professional will be able to explore dialectical behavior therapy (DBT) as a comprehensive treatment for severe and complex cases characterized by emotional dysregulation.

Chapter 7 introduces trial-based cognitive therapy (TBCT) as a transdiagnostic approach to broadening the reach of CBT, offering specific techniques to alter cognitions at each level.

Chapter 8 presents acceptance and commitment therapy (ACT) as a model for promoting psychological flexibility and behavior change across diagnostic categories.

Chapter 9 delves into metacognitive therapy (MCT) as an approach that focuses on cognition about cognition, targeting beliefs about thoughts and cognitive processes such as worry and rumination.

Chapter 10 explores compassion-focused therapy as a transdiagnostic intervention for self-criticism, offering techniques to nurture affiliative motivations and emotions.

In Chap. 11, the reader can examine the unified protocol (UP) approach for emotional disorders, highlighting its effectiveness in targeting transdiagnostic underlying cognitive and behavioral processes.

Chapter 12 addresses stress and burnout , discussing CBT interventions aimed at managing these pervasive issues across diagnostic boundaries.

Chapter 13 describe about Process-Based Therapy (PBT) that represents a new way of thinking, moving from diagnosis-driven interventions to an individualized treatment approach that recognizes the complexity of human suffering.

Last, but not least, Chap. 14 explores the application of CBT associated with pharmacotherapy for anxious and depressive disorders, offering a comprehensive approach to symptom management.

In general, this book addresses the main protocols of CBT in a single volume, offering practical insights and strategies for addressing emotional regulation and psychological distress. The contributions of experienced clinicians and therapists, as authors, ensure that readers have access to a diverse range of clinical practices and interventions. By emphasizing the importance of conceptualizing clients in their personal uniqueness, this book promotes a holistic approach to treatment that goes beyond traditional diagnostic labels.

In summary, this book offers a comprehensive overview of transdiagnostic approaches in cognitive behavioral therapy, providing clinicians and students with a wealth of techniques and interventions supported by empirical evidence. This book serves as a comprehensive guide to CBT and its transdiagnostic approaches, offering valuable insights and practical techniques for promoting emotional health and well-being in diverse populations. Whether you are a student learning about CBT or a seasoned professional seeking to enhance your practice, this book provides a wealth of information and resources to support your journey in the field of mental health and psychotherapy.

Finally, by presenting a range of CBT transdiagnostic protocols, this book equips readers with the tools they need to promote emotional health and well-being across diverse populations.

Current President of the Brazilian Federation of Cognitive Behavior Therapy—FBTC

Rio de Janeiro, Brazil — Angela Donato Oliva,

Contents

About the Contributors

Pricila Albrecht Bornholdt Licensed in Clinical Psychologist. Master's Degree in Psychology from the Postgraduate Program of Psychology at the Federal University of Santa Catarina (UFSC), Brazil. Specialist in Behavioral Analytical Clinic from the Núcleo Paradigma, Brazil. FAP (Functional Analytic Psychotherapy) Therapist FAP Trainer Certified from the FAP CEP Board Committee—USA. Experience in clinical area with an emphasis in Contextual Behavioral Therapies, especially FAP. Experience as a Professor in a University, Training and Specialization Courses in Clinical Behavioral Psychology FAP. Leader of the Global Project Live with Awareness, Courage and Love, created by Mavis Tsai. Affiliated with ACBS-Brazil (Brazilian Association for Contextual Behavioral Sciences) and ABPMC (Brazilian Association of Behavioral Sciences). Clinical Psychologist, Clinical Supervisor and Professor. Co-author of the "Baralho da FAP", published in Brazil, a therapeutic resource to do evocations in session and to enhance the therapeutic relationship.

Camilla Volpato Broering Licensed in Clinical Psychologist. Master's Degree and Doctoral's degree in Health Psychology, Psychosocial Processes and Psychological Development, with an emphasis on pre-surgical psychological preparation for children, from the Federal University of Santa Catarina (UFSC), Brazil. A Professor of the University in Psychology at the University of Vale do Itajaí (UNIVALI). Also, a Professor in Specialization and Postgraduate Courses in Psychology at various institutions throughout Brazil. Training in Cognitive-Behavioral Therapy and experience in the area of Cognitive-Behavioral interventions with children, adolescents and adults. Supervisor of clinical practice in Cognitive-Behavioral Therapy, a reviewer of scientific articles and the author of technical and Children's books. Certified Cognitive Behavior Therapist by FBTC (Brazilian Federation of Cognitive Therapies). Associate of AESBE (Association for Evidence-Based Teaching and Supervision). Member of the GT (working group) on Processes, Health and research from a cognitive-behavioral perspective of ANPEPP (National Association for Research and Postgraduate Studies in

Psychology). Co-author of the "Baralho da FAP", published in Brazil, a therapeutic resource to do evocations in session and to enhance the therapeutic relationship.

Katia Caetano Licensed as a Clinical psychologist and Professor in different Brazilian universities. Postdoctoral training at the East Bay Behavior Therapy Center, California, US. MS and PhD from University of São Paulo, Brazil. International fellowship at Boston University supervised by Prof. Stefan Hofmann, PhD, in the Psychotherapy and Emotion Research Laboratory/Boston University. MS in Psychobiology from University of São Paulo, Brazil. Supervisor and researcher of CBT and evidence-based treatments since 2010. Certified in Trial-based Cognitive Therapy (TBCT).

Ramiro Figueiredo Catelan Licensed in psychologist and clinical supervisor with experience treating adults with autism spectrum disorder, giftedness, ADHD, and borderline personality disorder. He holds a PhD in Social Psychology and has been trained in cognitive-behavioral therapy, dialectical behavior therapy, and evidence-based psychotherapy. Postdoc Researcher and the Head of the Center for Maladaptive Daydreaming and Emotion Dysregulation Research at the Institute of Psychiatry, Federal University of Rio de Janeiro, Brazil. He is a member of the International Consortium for Maladaptive Daydreaming Research (ICMDR). His current research project focuses on factors associated with maladaptive daydreaming and emotion dysregulation experiences.

Fernanda Coutinho Licensed as a Psychologist. PhD in Mental Health and Master's in Clinical Psychology in Federal University of Rio de Janeiro (UFRJ). Professor in CBT specialization at PUC-Rio and Coordinator of the Cognitive Therapy Service Center (CATC). Certified Therapist by the Brazilian Federation of Cognitive Therapies (FBTC).

Marcio Moreira da Silva Licensed as a Clinical psychologist in Brazil. Author and Organizer of Psychology and Education books. Work as a psychologist in CAPS (Basic Psychosocial Program). Bachelors in Psychology from Doutor Leao Sampaio University. Certified as a Cognitive Behavior Therapist from CBI of Miami, and Psychology Applied in Education from Regional do Cariri University.

Juliana Caversan de Barros Licensed as a Psychologist, master's and doctorate from the Institute of Psychology at the Federal University of Rio de Janeiro (UFRJ). Cognitive-Behavioral Therapist certified by the Brazilian Federation of Cognitive Therapies (FBTC), with a specialization in Acceptance and Commitment Therapy (ACT) from the Brazilian Center for Contextual Behavioral Science (CECONTE). Specialist in Stress Control Training at the Marilda Lipp Institute of Psychology and Stress Control. She holds Advanced Practicum certification in REBT from the Albert Ellis Institute, New York. Clinical supervisor and mentor in 2nd and 3rd generation Cognitive-Behavioral approaches, and creator of Psychological Flexibility Training in the Corporate Environment (TFP-C).

Irismar Reis de Oliveira Professor of Psychiatry at the Department of Mental Health and Neurosciences, Federal University of Bahia, Brazil. Developer of Trial-Based Cognitive Therapy.

Débora C. Fava PhD in Psychology from Unisinos with a period as a scholar visitor at Palo Alto University (CA/USA) and a Master's degree in Human Cognition from PUCRS. She is a postgraduate professor at the Specialization level in Cognitive-Behavioral Therapy (CBT) in childhood and adolescence at several institutions. Director of the VilaELO Institute-courses in mental health, in Porto Alegre. Specialist in CBT (WP) and Clinical Psychology (Federal Psychology Council), she has training in Child Behavior Management from Piedmont Virginia Community College (USA). Developer of the FAVA Program—Facilitating interaction with Students. Psychotherapist in a private practice, advising children's schools where she develops training and training for teachers on socio-emotional development and behavior management. Certified Therapist by the Brazilian Federation of Cognitive Therapies (FBTC). Book organizer and author of books and chapters in the area of CBT in the clinical and school context.

Bruno A. Franco is a psychiatrist graduated from UERJ. Professor of Psychiatry and Mental Health at Unigranrio University in Duque de Caxias—RJ.

Vitor Friary Founder of the Center for Mindfulness in Brazil. Licensed Psychologist and MSc in CBT and Mindfulness. Author of books and several chapters of books. Peer reviewed Trainer in Mindfulness-based Cognitive Therapy and current Accredited Member of the Access MBCT Registry.

Heitor Pontes Hirata Licensed in Psychology and specialization in Contextual Behavioral Therapies. PhD and Master's in Psychology from the Federal University of Rio de Janeiro. Psychologist in private practice, professor and supervisor of the postgraduate course in CBT applied to childhood and adolescence at the Pontifical Catholic University of Rio de Janeiro.

Jan Luiz Leonardi Licensed in Psychology from PUC-SP, specialization in Behavioral Therapy through Paradigm, training in Dialectical Behavior Therapy by Behavioral Tech, master's degree in Experimental Psychology: Behavior Analysis through PUC-SP and a PhD in Clinical Psychology from USP. He was vice president of the Brazilian Association of Psychology and Behavioral Medicine (ABPMC) in 2015–2016 and president of the Brazilian Association of Evidence-Based Psychology in 2022–2023. Clinical psychologist, supervisor and mentor of psychologists, coordinator of Specialization in Evidence-Based Practice in Clinical Psychology from InPBE (Institute of Evidence-Based Psychology).

Lucia Emmanoel Novaes Malagris Licensed as a Clinical Psychologist with a doctorate and post-doctorate in the field of health psychology with a specialty in the field of stress. Certified Therapist by the Brazilian Federation of Cognitive Therapies. Director of the Institute of Psychology and Stress Control in Rio de Janeiro.

Wilson Vieira Melo Registered clinical psychologist, certified as a Cognitive Behavior Therapist (FBTC), PhD in Psychology (Federal University of Rio Grande do Sul, Brazil/University of Virginia, U.S.) Masters in Clinical Psychology (PUC–RS, Brazil). Supervisor and Professor in Post Graduation in Dialectical Behavior Therapy (Vila ELO). Intensive Training in Dialectical Behavior Therapy (The Linehan Institute/Behavioral Tech). Former President of the Brazilian Federation of Cognitive Therapy (FBTC 2019-2021/2021-2023).

André Luiz Moreno Licensed in Psychology, Master in Psychology, Doctor in Mental Health. Specialist in CBT, with additional training in Schema Therapy. Cognitive Therapist certified by FBTC. Professor and Supervisor of training and specialization courses in TCC. Mental Health Consultant and Scientific Communicator on Anxiety.

Antonio Egidio Nardi Full Professor of Psychiatry, School of Medicine, Federal University of Rio de Janeiro, Brazil. Psychiatrist and Member of National Academy of Science, Brazil.

Ana Claudia Ornelas Licensed as a Clinical Psychologist with 31 years of experience in Brazil. Licensed in Mental Health and registered in Massachusetts (USA). Areas of expertise include education, research and clinical. Published several articles as first author; book organizer and author of chapters about Cognitive Behavior Therapy (CBT). Certified as a Cognitive Behavior Therapist by Brazilian Federation of Cognitive Therapies (FBTC). Masters in Sexology (UGF, Brazil) and PhD in Mental Health and International Researcher (Federal University of Rio de Janeiro, Brazil/Boston University/Massachusetts General Hospital, U.S.). Professor and coordinator at CBI of Miami specialization courses (Cognitive Behavior Therapy; Mindfulness and Sexuality Human).

Maria Amélia Penido Registered clinical psychologist in Brazil. Certified as a Trial Based in Cognitive Therapist and Cognitive Behavior Therapist. Author of the book "Amor na era digital". Masters in Psychology and PhD in Psychology from Federal University Rio de Janeiro. She is on the board as a Director of the Brazilian Federation of Cognitive Therapy (FBTC) and was former President of ATC-Rio. Therapy and is a researcher in the National Association of Cognitive Behavior Therapy. Areas of expertise include treatment of anxiety, mood, social skills trainer, group, education and supervisor of Cognitive Behavior Therapy.

Laiana A. Quagliato is a psychiatrist and serves as a Professor of Child and Adolescent Psychiatry at IPUB/UFRJ. She is also a permanent professor in the Psychiatry and Mental Health Program at UFRJ.

Luiz Fellipe Rocha Clinical Psychologist graduated at UERJ (Universidade do Rio de Janeiro). Doctor degree in Social Psychology (UERJ). He is Cognitive Behavior Therapist from PUC-RS (Pontificia Universidade Catolica—Rio Grande do Sul). Adjunct Professor at Centro Universitário Serra dos Órgãos (UNIFESO).

Veronica Andrea Santos Licensed in clinical psychologist. Specialist in Cognitive Behavioral Therapy. Professor of the Postgraduate Course in Cognitive Behavioral Therapy at PUC-Rio. She works as a teacher and clinical supervisor in extension and postgraduate courses. Training in Schema Therapy by Wainer/ISST. Specialization in Contextual Behavioral Therapies by FACEFI. Master and PhD in Mental Health IPUB-UFRJ. Researcher at the Virtual Reality Laboratory of the Panic and Respiratory Laboratory at IPUB/UFRJ.

Lucianne Jobim Valdivia Licensed in Clinical Psychologist. Specialist in Clinical Psychology (CRPRS). Master in Psychiatry and Behavioral Sciences (UFRGS), DBT Therapist member of DBT team Poa, Brazil.

Chapter 1
History of Cognitive Behavior Therapy: Emotional Regulation Achievement

Ana Claudia Ornelas and Marcio Moreira da Silva

Introduction

Cognitive-behavioral therapy (CBT) is an evidence-based approach that has been continuously evolving. At the beginning of the twentieth century, when the empirical bases of cognitive-behavioral approaches aimed at Charles Darwin's evolutionary theory, it was discovered that research with animal learning could be generalized to man. The continuity between the human species and that of other lower animals contributed and encouraged the conduct of experimental studies based on animal models for understanding human behavior for many years (Falcone, 2006; Lipp & Malagris, 2011; Barbosa & Borba, 2010).

According to Barbosa and Borba (2010), the term "behavioral therapy" was used to define the treatment of mental disorders based on the new therapeutic focus of learning theories. Initially, therapeutic techniques were based on the respondent conditioning model and were not yet effective to be a clinical approach, as they were more rigid and inadequate at addressing complaints related to mental health as a whole. Eysenck, H. (1987) pointed out that as a result of this, between the 60 s and 70 s, there was a certain disinterest in behaviorist theories, but there was a great demand for a psychotherapeutic approach focused on intervention with the aim of modifying human behavior, mainly with the use of the principles of operant conditioning and classical conditioning. The proposal was based on the reduction of neurotic symptoms and, for a long time, was considered the most scientific approach of the time. One of the biggest criticisms of behavioral therapy was due to the choice of techniques by therapists in a directive way, with the aim of modifying behavioral

A. C. Ornelas (✉)
Sunshine Therapy, Malden, MA, USA

M. M. da Silva
CEMED, Missao Velha, Brazil

A. C. Ornelas (ed.), *Transdiagnostic Approaches in Cognitive Behavioral Therapy*, https://doi.org/10.1007/978-3-031-63494-9_1

symptoms that were inadequate, based on the stimulus and response model (Eysenck, 1987; Kupfer et al., 2002; Morris et al., 2005).

There were several possibilities for treatment in the clinic with the emergence of the first wave of evidence-based therapy. Classical Behavioral Therapy was based on the theories of Pavlov and Skinner, and this approach aimed to identify and modify unwanted behaviors by increasing responses that became conditioned (Fresco, 2013; Thoma et al., 2015). From there, other treatments were emphasized as cutting-edge, for example, systematic exposure that was used to treat phobias (Kanfer & Saslow, 2002). Systematic desensitization was developed by Joseph Wolpe, and the technique involved gradual exposure by imagination and/or "in vivo" in the face of feared situations (from the least anxiety progressing to the greatest anxiety), helping patients overcome phobias and anxieties (Kanfer & Saslow, 2002; Barbosa & Borba, 2010). Later, Rational-Emotive Therapy, which Albert Ellis developed, was focused on the identification and modification of irrational thoughts that lead to negative emotions as a precursor form of cognitive-behavioral therapy (Barbosa & Borba, 2010; Fresco, 2013; Thoma et al., 2015).

With the advancement of science came the emergence of the second wave, cognitive therapy created in the 1960s/1970s by Aaron Beck (Beck & Fleming, 2021). Cognitive therapy had as a striking feature the central emphasis of cognitive and maladaptive structures in the origins of emotional problems. In this aspect, the main focus combined cognitive interventions with traditional behavioral principles to achieve a more effective and lasting improvement in individuals (Hayes et al., 1996; Meuret et al., 2012). According to Beck and Fleming (2021), cognitive therapy was initiated to treat other disorders, such as anxiety, personality disorders, substance use, and suicidal ideation. The theory became comprehensive and catered to the types of psychopathologies described in the DSM (Diagnostic and Statistical Manual of Mental Health). It provided the basis for treatment as well as methods to increase validity of theories, such as the efficacy and effectiveness of therapy. For each new condition, there were clinical observations to identify typical maladaptive beliefs associated with the criteria of characteristics of the related disorder. Through scales and instruments to assess these beliefs, the treatment protocol would be developed based on the conceptualization and restructuring of dysfunctional beliefs, thus applying the behavioral strategies for the associated disorders (Beck & Fleming, 2021).

For decades cognitive therapy has been evolving and gaining new therapists' adherents for treatments with promising results. The results of numerous randomized clinical trials have brought effective protocols to psychotherapists as well as contributions of new effective models that could be contemplated in CBT. This historical evolution in psychology was based on a predominantly philosophical perspective to a much more empirical approach, which started with the first-generation behavioral therapies, moving on to the second generation of cognitive-behavioral therapies, and contextual therapies as a third generation (Aldao & Nolen-Hoeksema, 2010; Hayes et al., 2013; Herbert et al., 2013). However, this trend is decreasing; with contextual therapies, or third-generation therapies, becoming increasingly common in clinical practice. The different types of contextual therapy are based on the current functional contextual philosophy, whose basis has applications in any area of human life (Schweizer et al., 2020).

Behavioral therapy, when it includes acceptance and mindfulness, represents another promising path (Hofmann, 2008; Hofmann & Asmundson, 2008; Hayes et al., 2012). The striking feature of approaches based on acceptance and mindfulness is a view that human suffering arises when individuals restrict their lives in the aim of escaping or avoiding immediate pain or discomfort—and this way of dealing with pain, results in great harm to their overall well-being. Thus, cognitive-behavioral therapies integrate with mindfulness, acceptance, and experiential interventions with traditional behavior principles to achieve improvements in the frequency and durability of new more effective and lasting skills (Hopkinson & Neuringer, 2003; Goldin et al., 2008; Hofmann, 2008). The challenge faced by the field of contextual approaches of cognitive-behavioral therapy is directed towards a broader scope, where it is essential to understand the conditions necessary to keep the individual healthy (Hayes et al., 1996, 2012; John & Gross, 2004).

Based on the studies of Hayes et al. (2013), the process of achieving emotional regulation becomes an objective in the protocols. Transdiagnostic, this skill can be developed and has brought about a significant change in the third-generation approaches of cognitive-behavioral therapy. Eventually, emotions influence attention, decision-making, memory, physiological responses, and social interactions. However, even though various possibilities of intra and interpersonal processes are shaped, emotions take ownership of changes, whether in intensity, duration, or frequency (John & Gross, 2004; Hofmann & Asmundson, 2008; Hayes et al., 2012, 2013). The ability to successfully regulate emotions is related to several important aspects underlying mood and anxiety disorders. For example, anxiety disorders, in addition to emotional symptoms such as avoidance sensations, overcompensation, and struggle, provoke various physical symptoms that hinder the person's functionality. These difficulties associated with emotion regulations impact human behavior in such an overwhelming way that the individual cannot cope with natural day-to-day situations, generating consequences that generalize because they understand that the situation is dangerous and that they are incapable of facing it (John & Gross, 2004; Hofmann & Asmundson, 2008; Aldao & Nolen-Hoeksema, 2010; Hayes et al., 2012, 2013). The timeline below represents the evolution of CBT as an evidence-based approach from the first to the third generation (Fig. 1.1).

First generation: Hans Eysenck, one of the precursors of Behavioral Therapy (Clinical Psychology), in the 1950s, focused on science, rationality, and objectivity. The principles based on learning theory and evolutionary basis (animal study) and the goal was to focus on behavior change/in the symptom. Eysenck (1987) proposed a personality theory based on biological factors, arguing that individuals inherit a type of nervous system that affects their ability to learn and adapt to the environment. The same author contributed to clinical psychology, discovering that there were a series of different personality traits that were revealed by the same responses, naming personality dimensions including extraversion, introversion, neuroticism, and psychoticism. Eysenck's personality theory is still

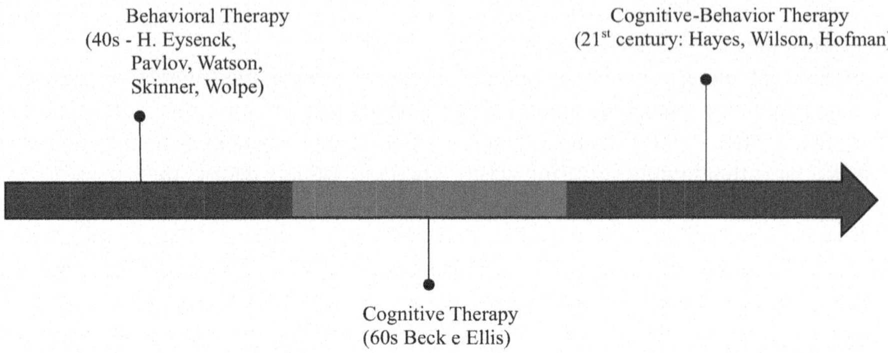

Fig. 1.1 Cognitive behavior-therapy evolution (twentieth to twenty-first century)

valid today to assess the tendencies of affects and well-being. Pavlov, and his theory with emphasis on objectivity, observed that the association of conditioned stimuli to neutral ones made them conditioned (Barbosa & Borba, 2010). Watson, through his experiments, created the theory of Social Modeling and Live Desensitization, which were later used in other research by Bandura and Wolpe to be applied in clinical psychology (Morris et al., 2005). Thorndike presented the concepts of the law of effect, where behavior could be reinforced and conditioned or punished to be extinct. Around the same time, Jacobson contributed a technique that is still widely used in therapy today, progressive muscle relaxation (Kanfer & Saslow, 2002). Morris et al. (2005) discuss that Skinner demonstrated behavioral therapy with radical behaviorism: the concept of *operant conditioning*, where behavior is conditioned with the increase in the frequency of a response through positive or negative reinforcements.

Second generation: Beck and Fleming (2021) describe that Aaron Beck began his studies with cognitive therapy in the 1960s, which showed that the emphasis on cognitive structures could result in psychological disorders. The central theme of cognitive therapy is the reconstruction of distorted beliefs. Albert Ellis presented rational emotive-behavioral therapy (REBT). In this approach, emotions and behaviors are based on the events and central/intermediate beliefs of individuals. Individuals interpret not the events themselves but understand situations through rigid and irrational generalization of beliefs.

Third generation: In transdiagnostic approaches, with highlights in Marsha Lineham's studies with DBT (Dialectical Behavior Therapy) and Steven Hayes with ACT (Acceptance and Commitment Therapy). The first, Dialectical Behavior Therapy (DBT) is a modified type of cognitive-behavioral therapy (CBT) and the main goals are to teach people to live in the moment, develop healthy ways to cope with stress, regulate their emotions, and improve their relationships with others (Chapman, 2006). DBT was originally planned to treat borderline personality disorder (BPD), but has been adapted to treat other mental health conditions beyond BPD. It can help people who have difficulty with emotional regulation or who exhibit self-destructive behaviors, such as eating disorders and substance use disorders (Chapman, 2006).

Acceptance and Commitment Therapy aims at psychological flexibility. The individual learns to identify, manage emotions with the aim of experiencing coping that enables self-regulation (Hofmann, 2008; Hayes et al., 2012, 2013). With scientific progress, a new idea about mental disorders arising from maladaptive beliefs was observed, for example, rumination which causes a tendency to repeatedly focus on the experience of negative emotion and its causes and consequences (Schweizer et al., 2020). The same authors demonstrate in their research that some individuals report rumination as a means of understanding the origins of their suffering, and this contradicts what studies by Zuzama et al. (2020) found about rumination, the results mean that it increases negative thinking congruent with mood, interfering with problem-solving and instrumental behavior, and distancing social support. In turn, rumination prospectively predicts symptoms and diagnoses of anxiety and depression (Lask et al., 2021).

The research by Zuzama et al. (2020) points out that cognitive strategies of emotional regulation and symptoms of four types of psychopathologies: depression, anxiety, eating disorders, and substance abuse. When multiple types of symptoms are gathered, mixed evidence of specificity in the relationship between emotional regulation strategies and psychopathology is found. Although all four strategies are significantly associated with psychopathology, the maladaptive strategies of rumination and suppression are more strongly associated with symptoms than the adaptive strategies of reappraisal and problem-solving (John & Gross, 2004). Outlining which strategies have stronger associations with psychopathology can help therapists identify those that play a more central role in the development, maintenance, and remission of various disorders (Hayes et al., 2013). This has implications for prevention programs that focus on the development of cognitive skills of emotional regulation, or even, treatments that focus on teaching regulatory skills may be targeted in prevention and intervention programs (Lask et al., 2021).

Lastly, to discuss emotional regulation, it is necessary to define what emotions are. James Gross, a researcher of emotions at Stanford University, sees emotions as brief responses that affect both behavior and the body, generated during events with potential to present challenges or opportunities (Gross, 1998). More importantly, he believes that emotions can be modulated or altered, and modulation is what determines the final emotional response.

Emotional regulation pertains to this modulation of emotion, in order to alter which emotions are experienced, as well as when and how they are experienced. The emotional regulation process model initiated by Gross (1998) details five main points of focus during emotional regulation: situation selection, situation modification, attention deployment, cognitive change, and response modification. While an individual is in a specific situation, they can also modify what they feel, and this is very relevant for unavoidable situations. In addition, a person can choose which specific aspects of the situation to focus on or selectively direct their attention or broaden their focus. The meaning an individual attributes to the event can also be modulated through cognitive change. How a person chooses to think about these situations, especially how she/he can rephrase or reassess her/his thinking in a more positive or adaptive way, is the focus of many types of contextual approaches based on cognitive-behavioral therapy. Most of the emotional regulation points proposed by this process model are focused on antecedent factors or occur before the emotional response. Table 1.1 represents the descriptions based on clinical strategies.

In conclusion, Gross (1998) specifically examined the difference between regulation strategies focused on antecedents and responses and found that although both methods were effective in reducing emotional expression, antecedent strategies (reassessment) were better at reducing the experience of emotion, while response strategies (suppression) induced physiological changes.

The approach is practical, where the therapist and the patient work collaboratively, promoting self-knowledge for better management of how to live their life. Here are some useful tips for everyday use:

- A good minute—at the beginning of a therapy session, or during a break between one client and another, take a 1-min break to breathe, have a tea or coffee, and visualize something that can bring self-care to the therapist and/or the client. Mindfulness and Meditation for example, are ways to regulate.
- In the face of a stressful or anxious situation, changing the temperature of the extremities can be helpful. Try removing shoes to feel the ground with your feet, running hands under water, listening to the noise of the water from the tap, or even focusing on the sounds in the environment around you. Looking around, try to describe the environment in detail.
- Throughout the body, breathe slowly, release the air deeply counting from 1 to 6 and inhale counting from 1 to 4, until you regulate your breathing and your heartbeat.
- Sit or lie down, breathe deeply and scan the whole body, part by part, let the weight of the body relax at each moment of this process.
- Count from 10 to 1, speaking words with gentle meanings between each count, such as peace, love, relief, well-being, balance.
- Professional Supervision: Regularly participate in supervisions for case discussion and professional support.

Table 1.1 Clinical strategies in CBT

Clinical strategies	Description
Emotional conscious	Recognize and understand the emotions that arise
Emotional acceptance	Allow oneself to feel different emotions without judgement
Emotional expression	Find healthy ways to express emotions
Emotional appraisal	Assess the validity of emotional responses to situations
Cognitive appraisal	Reframe thoughts to alter emotional response

Conclusion

The progress of cognitive-behavioral psychotherapies demonstrates a promise of a future based on a position where science transforms over the course of studies and, always, for the better in the field of mental health. What differentiates the application of cognitive-behavioral therapy is that the protocols address a form of structured, didactic therapy and are currently oriented towards each individual experience.

References

Aldao, A., & Nolen-Hoeksema, S. (2010). Specificity of cognitive emotion regulation strategies: A transdiagnostic examination. *Behaviour Research and Therapy, 48*(2010), 974–983.

Barbosa, J. C., & Borba, A. (2010). O surgimento das terapias cognitivo-comportamentais e suas consequências para o desenvolvimento de uma abordagem clínica analítico-comportamental dos eventos privados. *Revista Brasileira de Terapia Comportamental e Cognitiva, 12*(1–2), 60–79. http://pepsic.bvsalud.org/scielo.php?script=sci_arttext&pid=S1517-55452010000100004&lng=pt&tlng=pt

Beck, J. S., & Fleming, S. (2021, June 18). A brief history of Aaron T. Beck, MD, and cognitive behavior therapy. *Clinical Psychology in Europe, 3*(2), e6701. PMID: 36397957; PMCID: PMC9667129. https://doi.org/10.32872/cpe.6701.

Chapman, A. L. (2006). Dialectical behavior therapy: Current indications and unique elements. *Psychiatry (Edgmont), 3*(9), 62–68. PMID: 20975829; PMCID: PMC2963469.

Eysenck, H. (1987). Psychotherapy to behavior therapy: A paradigm shift. In D. B. Fishman, F. Rotgers, & C. Franks (Eds.), *Paradigms in behavior therapy: Present and promise*. Springer.

Falcone, E. M. O. (2006). As bases teóricas e filosóficas das abordagens cognitivo-comportamentais. Em: A. M. Jacó-Vilela; A. A. L. Ferreira & F. T. Portugal (Orgs.). *História da Psicologia. Rumos e percursos* (pp. 195–214). Rio de Janeiro: Nau Editora.

Fresco, D. M. (2013). Tending the garden and harvesting the fruits of behavior therapy. *Behavior Therapy, 44*(2), 177–179. https://doi.org/10.1016/j.beth. PMID: 23611067; PMCID: PMC4969569.

Goldin, P. R., McRae, K., Ramel, W., & Gross, J. J. (2008, March 15). The neural bases of emotion regulation: Reappraisal and suppression of negative emotion. *Biological Psychiatry, 63*(6), –577, 86. https://doi.org/10.1016/j.biopsych.2007.05.031. PMID: 17888411; PMCID: PMC2483789.

Gross, J. J. (1998). The emerging field of emotion regulation: An integrative review. *Review of General Psychology, 2*(3), 271–299. https://doi.org/10.1037/1089-2680.2.3.271

Hayes, S. C., Wilson, K. G., Gifford, E. V., Follette, V. M., & Strosahl, K. (1996). Experiential avoidance and behavioral disorders: A functional dimensional approach to diagnosis and treatment. *Journal of Consulting and Clinical Psychology, 64*, 1152–1168. [PubMed: 8991302].

Hayes, S. C., Strosahl, K. D., & Wilson, K. G. (2012). *Acceptance and commitment therapy: The process and practice of mindful change* (2nd ed.). Guilford Press.

Hayes, S. C., Levin, M. E., Plumb-Vilardaga, J., Villatte, J. L., & Pistorello, J. (2013). Acceptance and commitment therapy and contextual behavioral science: Examining the progress of a distinctive model of behavioral and cognitive therapy. *Behavior Therapy, 44*(2), 180–198. https://doi.org/10.1016/j.beth.2009.08.002. PMID: 23611068; PMCID: PMC3635495.

Herbert, J. D., Gaudiano, B. A., & Forman, E. M. (2013, December). The importance of theory in cognitive behavior therapy: A perspective of contextual behavioral science. *Behavior Therapy, 44*(4), 580–591. PMID: 24094783. https://doi.org/10.1016/j.beth.2013.03.001

Hofmann, S. G. (2008). Acceptance and commitment therapy: New wave or Morita therapy? *Clinical Psychology: Science and Practice, 15*, 280–285. https://doi.org/10.1111/j.1468-2850.2008.00138.x

Hofmann, S. G., & Asmundson, G. J. G. (2008). Acceptance and mindfulness-based therapy: New wave or old hat? *Clinical Psychology Review, 28*, 1–16. [PubMed: 17904260].

Hopkinson, J., & Neuringer, A. (2003). Modifying behavioral variability in moderately depressed students. *Behavior Modification, 27*, 251–264. [PubMed: 12705108].

John, O. P., & Gross, J. J. (2004). Healthy and unhealthy emotion regulation: Personality processes, individual difference, and life span development. *Journal of Personality, 72*, 1301–1333. [PubMed: 15509284].

Kanfer, F. H., & Saslow, G. (2002). Behavioral diagnosis. In C. M. Franks (Ed.), *Behavior therapy: Appraisal and status*. McGraw Hill.

Kupfer, D. J., First, M. B., & Regier, D. A. (Eds.). (2002). *A research agenda for DSM—V*. American Psychiatric Association.

Lask, L. S., Moyal, N., & Henik, A. (2021). Rumination, emotional intensity and emotional clarity. *Consciousness and Cognition, 96*, 103242. https://doi.org/10.1016/j.concog.2021.103242. Epub 2021 Nov 19. PMID: 34808490.

Lipp, M. E. N., & Malagris, L. E. N. (2011). Estresse: aspectos históricos, teóricos e clínicos. In B. Rangé (Org.), Psicoterapias cognitivo-comportamentais: um diálogo com a psiquiatria (pp.617–632). Porto Alegre: Artmed.

Meuret, A. E., Wolitzky-Taylor, K. B., Twohig, M. P., & Craske, M. G. (2012). Coping skills and exposure therapy in panic disorder and agoraphobia: Latest advances and future directions. *Behavior Therapy, 43*(2), 271–284. https://doi.org/10.1016/j.beth.2011.08.002. PMID: 22440065; PMCID: PMC3327306.

Morris, E. K., Smith, N. G., & Altus, D. E. B. F. (2005). Skinner's contributions to applied behavior analysis. *Behavior Analyst, 28*(2), 99–131. https://doi.org/10.1007/BF03392108. PMID: 22478444; PMCID: PMC2755377.

Schweizer, T. H., Snyder, H. R., Young, J. F., & Hankin, B. L. (2020). The breadth and potency of transdiagnostic cognitive risks for psychopathology in youth. *Journal of Consulting and Clinical Psychology, 88*(3), 196–211. https://doi.org/10.1037/ccp0000470

Thoma, N., Pilecki, B., & McKay, D. (2015). Contemporary cognitive behavior therapy: A review of theory, history, and evidence. *Psychodynamic Psychiatry, 43*(3), 423–461. https://doi.org/10.1521/pdps.2015.43.3.423. PMID: 26301761.

Zuzama, N., Fiol-Veny, A., Roman-Juan, J., & Balle, M. (2020). Emotion regulation style and daily rumination: Potential mediators between affect and both depression and anxiety during adolescence. *International Journal of Environmental Research and Public Health, 17*(18), 6614. https://doi.org/10.3390/ijerph17186614. PMID: 32932821; PMCID: PMC7559268.

Chapter 2
Transdiagnostic Approaches

Ana Claudia Ornelas and Marcio Moreira

Introduction

According to recent publications in psychology, traditional diagnostic systems may no longer be convenient for classifying mental illnesses, so for understanding the underlying biopsychosocial and clinical processes, transdiagnostic approaches could be more comprehensive than specific treatments (Fusar-Poli et al., 2019). Due to their potential, "transdiagnostic" approaches have possibilities to better represent the clinical and scientific reality regarding the evaluation criteria in mental health, in the context of complexity, dimensionality and comorbidity that is the norm in this clinical practice (Gros et al., 2017).

For many years, the Diagnostic and Statistical Manual of Mental Disorders, which is now in its 5th edition (DSM-5 TR) and the International Classification of Diseases (ICD 11) have achieved a global reach and still exert a profound influence on the ways in which metal disorders are understood, evaluated, and managed (APA, 2022; Mansell, 2019; Masyn et al., 2018). And yet, despite the widespread influence on the diagnostic hypothesis, there is an emerging and growing consensus that such psychiatric evaluations may be reaching the limits of their research and utility in the clinic, giving way to a "transdiagnostic" approach that goes beyond traditional diagnostic boundaries or, more radically, leaves them aside in general, to provide new insights on how people understand mental health difficulties (Waszczuk et al., 2018).

In this way, the professional realizes that in addition to diagnostic issues, the individuality of the person becomes more relevant, as it modifies the distinctions

A. C. Ornelas (✉)
Sunshine Therapy, Malden, MA, USA

M. Moreira
CEMED, Missao Velha, Brazil

A. C. Ornelas (ed.), *Transdiagnostic Approaches in Cognitive Behavioral Therapy*, https://doi.org/10.1007/978-3-031-63494-9_2

between the psychiatric disease proposed at the classification level and makes professionals aware of a new way of conceptualizing the theories and underlying processes involved in mental health problems, thus providing a platform for new focuses of thought on the onset, maintenance, clinical treatment, and progress related to experiences of disabling mental suffering.

History of the DSM—(APA)

Some of the history about the classification of mental health stands out, where only the diagnostic hypothesis when formalized appropriately as it arose from the biological and botanical classification systems of Linnaen of the nineteenth century. The most famous from the onset was Kraepelin's Compendium der Psychiatrie in 1883 (Compton & Guze, 1995). This was published in the United States, serving mainly as a basis for the first edition of the DSM in 1952 (DSM-I, American Psychiatric Association, 1980).

In fact, the model of the first DSM was based on the same source that investigates the origins of medical diseases, especially the discovery of bacteria as a source of infectious diseases (DSM-I, American Psychiatric Association, 1980). What caught attention at that time was the research being developed to identify the neurological causes of diseases, for example, separating dementia from other psychiatric diseases based on biological indicators (Compton & Guze, 1995). The same authors highlighted a greater advance in research on the concept that mental illness could have a biological basis and thus they would organize the structure of the criteria of psychiatric disorders based on patterns of characteristic symptoms researched within the observation of patients.

Psychiatry was recognized for the first time as a medical specialty in the United States by the Association of Medical Superintendents of American Institutions for the Insane. This organization became the American Psychiatric Association (APA) in 1921. (Moldawsky, 2020). The same author also mentioned that, between the 1940s and 1960s, American psychiatry was heavily influenced by psychoanalytic theory. During this period, American psychiatry emphasized individual differences rather than commonalities in diseases. The mental processes of health and psychological illness were considered similar. However, the lack of a unified and biological classification system for psychiatric diseases progressed even with psychiatry contradicting the entire scientific context compared to the rest of medicine. Psychoanalysis ended up being exhausted and attacked in American psychiatry with the discovery of psychiatric drugs that were increasingly used for the treatment of severe psychiatric diseases. Additionally, the emergence of scientific research based on the biology of mental disorders surfaced with important findings about the influence of neurotransmitter systems (Mansell, 2019).

The United States took the initiative to create a diagnostic manual, which described 21 disorders, where 19 were psychotic disorders, but this was set aside by American psychiatrists in 1942 (Waszczuk et al., 2018). Later between 1952 and

1968, the American Psychiatric Association released the first two versions of its diagnostic criteria for psychiatric disorders, but diagnostic reliability and validity would only be established decades later (APA, 1987). It was not until 1970 that a prominent study involving researchers from the USA and the UK illustrated the importance of having a unified diagnostic system to determine the prevalences of psychiatric diseases (APA, 1987).

A study was conducted to clarify large discrepancies reported between the statistics of the USA (New York) and the UK (London) on the proportions of adults with hospital admissions for schizophrenia and manic-depressive disease (APA, 1980; Compton & Guze, 1995). Using semi-structured interviews, video tape classifications, and systematic examination of case records, the study found that diagnostic methods were inconsistent for routine hospital admissions among the sites responsible for patient screenings and diagnostic discrepancies occurred. Many of the patients diagnosed with schizophrenia in New York, for example, would have been diagnosed with manic-depressive disease in London (Masyn et al., 2018).

Diagnostic agreement would not be possible until reliable diagnostic systems emerged, such as the DSM-III in 1980 (APA, 1980; Masyn et al., 2018). Biopsychosocial processes consider the interaction of underlying biological, psychological, and social factors in understanding health and disease. These are the processes that are included in transdiagnostic approaches. Perhaps an unintended consequence of psychiatric diagnosis is the notion that diagnoses somehow capture or reflect the underlying reality of the world, observing the nature of symptoms in their common characteristics and identifying the types of symptoms related to mental disorder in a generalized way. This idea comes from general medicine, where most physical and emotional diseases reflect qualitatively different health states, with one or even a small number of identifiable and discrete causes (McEvoy et al., 2009; Markon et al., 2011).

Studies show that mental illness prototypically emerges from an interaction between biological, behavioral, psychosocial, and cultural aspects. However, these aspects are not always included in established diagnoses where interactions are multiple and modulated by subjective and individual experiences throughout life (Dalgleish et al., 2020). Dalgleish et al. (2020) addresses other factors in their studies, such as the issue of comorbidity of criteria in psychiatry. An example of this is when someone presents one or more conditions of emotional or physical problems that meet the criteria for more than one diagnosis at the same time. As long as there is an understanding of comorbidities, it would not be a problem for the diagnostic model. However, what is concerning is that the Epidemiological findings reveal that comorbidity among psychiatric diagnoses is the rule, not the exception. To conceptualize a clinical case of a single and uncomplicated group of symptoms would, in fact, be relatively scarce (Dalgleish et al., 2020; Van Loo & Romeijn, 2015).

The greatest severity would still be associated with functional impairment and also quality of life, for example, the chronicity of symptoms leading the individual to greater difficulty in their overall functionality (Van Loo & Romeijn, 2015). For a long time, mental health professionals relied on a central question of diagnostic compendiums seeking to conceptualize which symptoms to include to delineate a certain disorder. This was complex given that many symptoms of mental health problems would also be characteristics of everyday life, for example, fatigue, bad mood, and lack of motivation being associated with a multiplicity of signs and symptoms. In the case of depression, for example, which again provides a revealing illustration with established measurement tools and accesses, there are about 280 different instruments developed in the last century, many of which are still in use (Santor et al., 2006). These instruments differ in the assessment of the signs and symptoms they describe as common in depression. Notwithstanding the fact that some of these 280 instruments may have weak clinical validity, as there is a vast range of clinical signs and symptoms that are identified in the instruments. This suggests that there is not a single set of symptoms that define depression (and, by extension, other diagnostic categories) and consequently, the profile outlined in diagnostic manuals may be excessively narrow or rigid.

Studies focused on identifying and classifying conditions based on specific criteria for diagnosis may be failing to reasonably capture the factors that cross categories beyond clinical data (Borsboom, 2017; Borsboom & Cramer, 2013). While diagnostic approaches are specific, transdiagnostic ones are more comprehensive and consider treatments that can be applied to different disorders in different individuals. Though the vision of transdiagnostic approaches seemingly changes the course in observing the symptoms of mental illness, it encompasses a model that respects different components of the emotional dimension (Borsboom, 2017; Borsboom & Cramer, 2013).

Research on transdiagnostic treatments in emotional disorders has increased in the last 15 years, with a notable increase in the number of clinical trials evaluating scientific evidence of these treatments. Several advantages have been attributed to transdiagnostic treatments, most notably is the ability to address multiple emotional disorders using the same treatment protocol.

Thus, treatment can be more economical and mental health professionals only need to be trained in one protocol that addresses various psychological problems. Secondly, training professionals in a treatment approach, rather than a different protocol for each emotional disorder, can facilitate the dissemination of evidence-based treatments for these specific problems. This approach may be of particular interest in ecological settings such as public services, where mental health professionals have to treat patients with heterogeneous diagnostic presentations where difficulty comes in appropriate selection of protocols, therapeutic techniques, or even the definition of a single treatment as a common denominator for the intervention of all symptoms outlined in emotional disorders. The third important advantage is that comorbid mental disorders can be more appropriately targeted because these protocols generally focus on what these disorders have in common, not on variations of specific disorder symptoms.

For example, extensive research shows the fundamental role played by neuroticism in the onset and maintenance of both anxiety disorders and depressive disorders, indicating its relevance in research and clinical practice. In this sense, the "shared mechanisms approach", described by Sauer-Zavala et al. (2017), is based on the assumption that there are underlying central mechanisms related to anxiety disorders. Comorbidity in emotional disorders has been associated with greater severity and impairment, poorer quality of life, and disease chronicity. However, the effective use of strategies is not well supported by existing empirical evidence (McManus et al., 2010).

Hirsch et al. (2021) reported that the most appropriate approach to dealing with comorbidity would be the application of treatments based on a transdiagnostic perspective, although this term has been used to refer to different approaches to emotional problems. Based on these approaches, some authors have argued that a transdiagnostic treatment may be appropriate for a wide range of disorders, including all anxiety and unipolar mood disorders, and even somatoform and dissociative disorders, while facilitating the treatment of patients with comorbidities (McManus et al., 2010; Sauer-Zavalla et al., 2017; Talkovsky et al., 2017).

However, there are other transdiagnostic approaches to the treatment of emotional disorders (including the treatment of comorbid presentations), such as Dialectical Behavior Therapy or "third wave" therapies (for example, mindfulness and acceptance and commitment therapy).

As in cases, for example, where the person complains of difficulty concentrating, fatigue, and insomnia, one symptom may simply interfere with the other. If the choice of the proposal is diagnostic, it would be in the attempt to assess the duration of these symptoms, where the therapist could create a hierarchy in the intervention of the most severe symptoms to the least severe and frame these symptoms in a disorder already existing in the mental health statistics manual (Dalgleish et al., 2020; Hofmann, 2014). This would be different from the view of transdiagnostic approaches, where it would conceptualize predisposition, environment, and self-regulation skills, performing a more holistic intervention (Hofmann, 2014).

On the other hand, the field of mental health has witnessed a great growth of intervention and implementation research to address mental health problems in various aspects, such as cultural, social, psychological, and biological influence (Masyn et al., 2018). Emotional disorders are common mental health conditions and one of the main causes of suffering and impairment worldwide.

Finally, transdiagnostic approaches have the potential to address "otherwise unspecified" (NOS) diagnoses, for which there are still no evidence-based treatments in the literature and with an increase in research and publications on the effectiveness of transdiagnostic treatment, it is assumed that new research based on these unspecified conditions will soon come (Gonzalez-Robles et al., 2018). At the moment, several meta-analyses have demonstrated the effectiveness of these treatments in adults with emotional disorders, compared to control conditions, in measures of general anxiety and specific anxiety, as well as depression and quality of life (Gonzalez-Robles et al., 2018; Masyn et al., 2018).

In a meta-analysis on the effectiveness of these protocols, compared to CBT for single disorders, they found no significant differences in the effectiveness of these two treatment approaches for anxiety. In order to examine how comorbidity can be related and evaluated in clinical trials that analyze transdiagnostic protocols, the importance of comorbidity aspects such as clinical severity, clinical course, and frequency in patients with comorbid anxiety and depressive disorders is emphasized

(Talkovsky et al., 2017). Some studies on transdiagnostic treatments for emotional disorders have evaluated the effects of treatment on comorbid symptoms, as well as on main symptoms (Fusar-Poli et al., 2019; Dalgleish et al., 2020).

More recently, Moldawsky (2020) studied a significant advancement in the integration of measures in clinical trials. The study described a multimodal investigation based on individual differences in a variable process called attentional control. This process presented clinical responses in the context of a brief transdiagnostic treatment for anxiety and depression. Hirsch et al. (2021) described an example of clinical translation of basic science about the negative interpretation bias of affective aspects. The same researchers found that increasing interpretation training for repetitive negative thinking could generate positive results. Images facilitated interpretations of more positive emotional factors reduced intrusions of thoughts, attention and, after training, there was a reduction in rumination.

Mansell (2019) observed that when modeling individual processes, as well as general processes in individuals with borderline personality disorder, he found a significant degree of heterogeneity in interpersonal relationships and affective domains.

Research on transdiagnostic and cognitive-behavioral intervention compared to the standard of previous treatments and usual care for treating people with severe irritability, show surprising and significant results regarding the treated attentional focus (Dagleish et al., 2020; Andrews et al., 2018).

Finally, studies on transdiagnostic approaches define some standards for treatment to be evidence-based and can continue the research to determine a better prognosis in the context of mental health (González-Robles et al., 2018).

Table 2.1 summarizes the transdiagnostic approaches containing the various clinical interventions that will be presented in the chapters of this book.

Clinical Case

C., female, now 26 years old, single and without a steady relationship currently. In her life story, she says that she was raised in a home with strict education, a very cold father and the house rules had to be followed. C. started dating her first husband L. when she was 16 years old. One day, C. and L. were thrown out on the street and C.'s father found out that they were already sexually involved, as C.'s parents were very religious, they asked her and her boyfriend to leave home and get married to maintain a clean life under God's laws. C. and L. got married, but everything was very difficult, C. was unable to study and worked as a nanny to survive. At work she could eat and still have a small salary, but life was very restricted at that time. One day she came home early and found a plate of white flour on the table, not knowing what it was, she threw it away. Later, she understood that the flour was a drug (cocaine) that her husband used.

Upon discovering that her husband was a drug user, she asked him to stop the addiction, and since then, a nightmare began in her life. L., upon realizing that she

Table 2.1 Transdiagnostic approaches and biopsychosocial models

Transdiagnostic approaches—CBT	Biopsychosocial model
Trial based in cognitive behavior therapy	This method encourages a more profound therapeutic change across a wide spectrum of mental health disorders
Unified protocol	Given the significant rates of comorbidity encountered in clinical practice, the notion of formulating and intervening with transdiagnostic underlying cognitive and behavioral processes has become the subject of increasing attention
Mindfulness based in cognitive behavioral therapy	Mindfulness and acceptance-based cognitive behavioral psychotherapies offer a systematic approach to understanding human suffering, and view processes such as experiential avoidance, cognitive fusion, and rumination for example as central elements in the maintenance of psychological distress
Dialectical behavior therapy	DBT intervention works as a tool for the treatment of severe and complex cases, where emotional dysregulation leads the individual to behave in a maladaptive way
Functional analytic therapy	FAP is a third-generation approach from CBT that uses the therapeutic relationship as a strategy to promote more effective interpersonal and intimacy repertoires
Stress and burnout	Transdiagnostic brings together approaches with proven evidence and effective strategies to meet these demands, develop psychological flexibility, promote behavioral changes, and rescue the quality of life of the affected individuals
Compassion focused therapy	To access and nurture their affiliative motivations, emotions, and competencies, which can be part of the compassionate self-experience
Acceptance and commitment therapy	ACT combines acceptance and attention processes with commitment and behavior change processes to create psychological flexibility
Process-based therapy	The integration with genetics, evolutionary psychology, neurosciences and other areas of knowledge can mutually contribute, to move towards the practice of what really works
Metacognitive	To propose an increase in attentional flexibility, that means it changes in how people return to their attention to thoughts at first moment that are just events present in consciousness
Medication and CBT treatment	To discuss treatment proposals associating CBT and pharmacotherapy with the intention of better controlling and stabilizing the severe symptoms of anxiety and depression

was throwing his cocaine away, dragged her by the hair and said that now she could only leave the house when he allowed. She lived for 5 years imprisoned by her husband, going hungry, and suffering from her husband's mood swings; she couldn't even visit her family. In addition to being forced to abort two pregnancies, she was forced to take solutions to cause the abortion. C. managed to leave home with the help of an aunt who lived in another region; she moved and restarted her life. C. is 26 years old and, after being psychologically evaluated, presented criteria for unipolar mood disorder, compulsive eating disorder, post-traumatic stress, panic disorder and agoraphobia. She uses fluoxetine 20 mg, the medication prescribed by the

Table 2.2 Pros and cons to promote the client's motivation for treatment

Motivational questions—pros and cons
•"What would you like to be different in your current situation?"
• "What makes you think you need to change?"
• "What happens if you don't change?"
• "What will be different if you complete your goal and achieve what you want this next week?"
• "What would be the advantages of changing your food-related habits?"
• "What would your life be like in 2 years if you continued to be motivated in this therapeutic plan?"
• "What makes you think that others are concerned about your well-being?"
• "How can I help you overcome some of the difficulties you are facing?"
• "If you decided to change, what would you have to do to make it happen?"
• "Suppose you don't change, what's the WORST thing that could happen?"
• "What is the BEST thing you could imagine that could come out of change?"

psychiatrist. C. still has difficulties in starting and maintaining a school or professional activity, has low socio-emotional functionality and few friends. In the anamnesis, some motivational questions were asked and later the pros and cons were outlined in relation to the changes that C. outlined as goals.

One first step is represented in Table 2.2; the clinician can address the client's motivation for the therapeutic process using some questions that can help to reflect on the advantages and disadvantages of changing.

From there, a treatment plan was carried out with the following steps: psychoeducation techniques, guided discovery, rational-emotive behavioral therapy, mindfulness, and exposure. C. managed to motivate herself for the treatment and successfully carried out the steps of this protocol. Today, after 8 months of treatment, C. is emotionally involved with a stable boyfriend, preparing to enter a higher education course in Pedagogy and, feeling more confident and more aware of her emotions. She still has memories of her story, but every day, she sets her intentions and goals, while being kind to herself. This strengthens her in her presentations and in her emotional growth daily.

Conclusion

Finally, the main basis for progress in this context would allow the development of a relevant theory, where the transdiagnostic field is based on theoretical foundations, especially in working on central processes and nosology, as well as enabling mental health professionals to understand the individual aspects that differentiate the specific diagnosis to the processes and factors inherent to personality. Addressing important and functional issues in the clinical area in the individualization of treatment would be the ideal focus.

References

American Psychiatric Association. (1980). *Diagnostic and statistical manual of mental disorders* (3rd ed.). American Psychiatric Association.

American Psychiatric Association. (1987). *Diagnostic and statistical manual of mental disorders* (3rd ed., rev.). American Psychiatric Association.

American Psychiatric Association. (2022). *Diagnostic and statistical manual of mental disorders* (5th ed., text rev.). American Psychiatric Association. https://doi.org/10.1176/appi.books.9780890425787

Andrews, G., Basu, A., Cuijpers, P., Craske, M. G., McEvoy, P. M., English, C. L., & Newby, J. M. (2018). Computer therapy for the anxiety and depression disorders is effective, acceptable and practical health care: An updated meta-analysis. *Journal of Anxiety Disorders, 55*, 70–78.

Borsboom, D. (2017). A network theory of mental disorders. *World Psychiatry, 16*, 5–13. https://doi.org/10.1002/wps.20375

Borsboom, D., & Cramer, A. O. J. (2013). Network analysis: An integrative approach to the structure of psychopathology. *Annual Review of Clinical Psychology, 9*, 91–121.

Compton, W. M., & Guze, S. B. (1995). The neo-Kraepelinian revolution in psychiatric diagnosis. *European Archives of Psychiatry and Clinical Neuroscience, 245*(4–5), 196–201. https://doi.org/10.1007/BF02191797

Dalgleish, T., Black, M., Johnston, D., & Bevan, A. (2020). Transdiagnostic approaches to mental health problems: Current status and future directions. *Journal of Consulting and Clinical Psychology, 88*(3), 179–195. https://doi.org/10.1037/ccp0000482

Fusar-Poli, P., Solmi, M., Brondino, N., Davies, C., Chae, C., Politi, P., Borgwardt, S., Lawrie, S. M., Parnas, J., & McGuire, P. (2019). Transdiagnostic psychiatry: A systematic review. *World Psychiatry, 18*(2), 192–207. https://doi.org/10.1002/wps.20631

González-Robles, A., Díaz-García, A., Miguel, C., García-Palacios, A., & Botella, C. (2018). Comorbidity and diagnosis distribution in transdiagnostic treatments for emotional disorders: A systematic review of randomized controlled trials. *PLoS One, 13*(11), e0207396. https://doi.org/10.1371/journal.pone.0207396. PMID: 30440020; PMCID: PMC6237379.

Gros, D. F., Szafranski, D. D., & Shead, S. D. (2017). A real world dissemination and implementation of Transdiagnostic Behavior Therapy (TBT) for veterans with affective disorders. *Journal of Anxiety Disorders, 46*, 72–77. https://doi.org/10.1016/j.janxdis.2016.04.010. Epub 2016 Apr 27. PMID: 27158076.

Hirsch, J., Tiede, M., Zhang, X., Noah, J. A., Salama-Manteau, A., & Biriotti, M. (2021). Interpersonal agreement and disagreement during face-to-face dialogue: An fNIRS investigation. *Frontiers in Human Neuroscience, 14*, 601. https://doi.org/10.3389/fnhum.2020.606397

Hofmann, S. G. (2014). *The Wiley handbook of cognitive behavioral therapy*. Wiley Blackwell/Wiley.

Mansell, W. (2019). Transdiagnostic psychiatry goes above and beyond classification. *World Psychiatry, 18*, 360–361. https://doi.org/10.1002/wps.20680

Markon, K. E., Chmielewski, M., & Miller, C. J. (2011). The reliability and validity of discrete and continuous measures of psychopathology: A quantitative review. *Psychological Bulletin, 137*, 856–879. https://doi.org/10.1037/a0023678

Masyn, K. E., Henderson, C. E., & Greenbaum, P. E. (2018). Exploring the latent structures of psychological constructs in social development using the dimensional-categorical spectrum. *Social Development, 12*, 82–86.

McEvoy, P. M., Nathan, P., & Norton, P. J. (2009). Efficacy of transdiagnostic treatments: A review of published outcome studies and future research directions. *Journal of Cognitive Psychotherapy, 23*, 20–33. https://doi.org/10.1891/0889-8391.23.1.20

McManus, F., Shafran, R., & Cooper, Z. (2010). What does a transdiagnostic approach have to offer the treatment of anxiety disorders? *British Journal of Clinical Psychology, 49*, 491–505. https://doi.org/10.1348/014466509X476567

Moldawsky, R. J. (2020). Is the psychiatric history losing its relevance? *The Permanente Journal, 24*, 19.186. https://doi.org/10.7812/TPP/19.186

Santor, D. A., Gregus, M., & Welch, A. (2006). Eight decades of measurement in depression. *Measurement: Interdisciplinary Research and Perspectives, 4*(3), 135–155. https://doi.org/10.1207/s15366359mea0403_1

Sauer-Zavala, S., Cassiello-Robbins, C., Conklin, L. R., Bullis, J. R., Thompson-Hollands, J., & Kennedy, K. A. (2017). Isolating the unique effects of the unified protocol treatment modules using single case experimental design. *Behavior Modification, 41*(2), 286–307. https://doi.org/10.1177/0145445516673827. Epub 2016 Oct 22. PMID: 28198196.

Talkovsky, A. M., Green, K. L., Osegueda, A., & Norton, P. J. (2017). Secondary depression in transdiagnostic group cognitive behavioral therapy among individuals diagnosed with anxiety disorders. *Journal of Anxiety Disorders, 46*, 56–64. https://doi.org/10.1016/j.janxdis.2016.09.008. Epub 2016 Sep 28. PMID: 27707524.

Van Loo, H. M., & Romeijn, J. W. (2015). Psychiatric comorbidity: Fact or artifact? *Theoretical Medicine and Bioethics, 36*(1), 41–60. https://doi.org/10.1007/s11017-015-9321-0. PMID: 25636962; PMCID: PMC4320768.

Waszczuk, M. A., Zimmerman, M., Ruggero, C., Li, K., MacNamara, A., Weinberg, A., et al. (2018). What do clinicians treat: Diagnoses or symptoms? The incremental validity of a symptom-based, dimensional characterization of emotional disorders in predicting medication prescription patterns. *Comprehensive Psychiatry, 79*, 80–88. https://doi.org/10.1016/j.comppsych.2017.04.004

Chapter 3
The Importance of Case Conceptualization and Therapeutic Alliance

Ana Claudia Ornelas and Marcio Moreira da Silva

Introduction

To understand the content of this chapter, it is necessary to describe the concept of transdiagnostic, which can be defined as the transpositions of symptoms or also the non-specificity of characteristics that close only one diagnosis in mental disorders (Johansson et al., 2012; Sauer-Zavala et al., 2017; Steele et al., 2018). Among transdiagnostic patients, more than one hypothesis can be conceptualized in relation to emotional disorders of anxiety and mood. Currently, it is common to evaluate a patient who presents a variety of symptoms that lead to various diagnostic frames (Barlow et al., 2011).

Studies show that when performing the evaluation and clinical conceptualization, the mental health professional can intervene with greater evidence both in adherence and in the patient's response to treatment (Barlow et al., 2011; Johnston et al., 2011; Steele et al., 2018). Both psychotherapy and psychiatry, with the aim of making their practices more scientific, use case conceptualization as a first step to obtain a good prognosis in treatment.

Conceptualization allows the therapist a guide through scientific instruments such as interviews, anamneses, scales and/or inventories, thus achieving better foundations and bases for a favorable prognosis in psychological treatment (Kotov et al., 2017; Lambert, 2013). The objectives of this chapter consist of describing the concepts and scientifically grounding the transdiagnostic protocols in the literature.

A. C. Ornelas (✉)
Sunshine Therapy, Malden, MA, USA

M. M. da Silva
CEMED, Missao Velha, Brazil

A. C. Ornelas (ed.), *Transdiagnostic Approaches in Cognitive Behavioral Therapy*, https://doi.org/10.1007/978-3-031-63494-9_3

The New Variation of Psychiatry in the Transdiagnostic Approach

Regarding the epidemiology of transdiagnostic, the prevalence of 25% of individuals with anxiety and mood disorders is estimated (Andrade et al., 2012). Based on this data, it is observed that in the general population there is a trend towards greater awareness of the need for treatment of these clinical conditions. These diagnoses present potential disadvantages of the functionality and productivity. Examples include individuals who have diagnoses of depression, social anxiety, or panic disorder, who have great difficulties in carrying out their social activities and professions regularly (Aldao & Nolen-Hoeksema, 2010; Andrade et al., 2012; Zitman, 2012).

The removal of distinctions between the psychiatric proposal at the level of classification in the International Code of Diseases (ICD-11) and in the Manual of Mental Health Statistics (DSM-5) allows for new ways of classifying mental health problems. New conceptualizations and alternatives of processes linked with mental health begin to emerge, and with this, a platform for new ways of thinking about the onset, maintenance, and clinical treatment as well as the recovery from experiences of debilitating mental suffering. Even though there are people who do not meet any diagnostic hypothesis criteria, they may also suffer at some point in life, with emotional intensity, frequency, and durability that hinder their functioning (Kotov et al., 2017; Sauer-Zavala et al., 2017; Schweizer et al., 2020). Support and backing for a transdiagnostic approach surpasses the traditional limits of diagnosis or, assertively, sets them aside, and provides new models of conceptualization and understanding about the difficulties of the individual who suffers from any emotional disorder (Brown & Barlow, 2002; Cape et al., 2010; DeOrnelasMaia et al., 2013, 2015).

The transdiagnostic field is still a very new concept, however, it is rapidly developing. The breadth of ambition varies between dimensional approaches to guide clinical evaluation, and to carry out the intervention (DeOrnelasMaia et al., 2015; Kraus et al., 2011; Ruggero et al., 2019) and accommodate characteristics arising from personality, as well as development trajectories, including cognitive risk dimensions (Monteiro, 2010; Kotov et al., 2017; Schweizer et al., 2020). However, more formal approaches were a bit more restricted in responses or symptoms (Craddock & Owen, 2010).

Clinical Conceptualization

CBT, being an evidence-based approach, highlights as therapy objectives (1) to assess the intervening variables (predisposing and maintaining factors) that interfere with problematic behaviors; (2) to understand together with the client what he/she considers to be functional and dysfunctional behaviors and; (3) to plan treatment and prevent relapses. Still in the same proposal, CBT enables the establishment of goals, through which are identified the testable automatic thoughts that prevent the achievement of these goals. The frequency of these thoughts is mutually assessed by the therapist and client during the sessions, through guided discovery, using questions related to the evidence of the affirmations and conclusions that the client establishes in the face of the facts that occur in client's day-to-day life (Kotov et al., 2017; Lambert, 2013; Marçal, 2005).

During the anamnesis, where the collection of information about the client is carried out, the therapist by being comprehensive, empathetic, and trustworthy will favor the engagement and return of the client for subsequent sessions. The continuity of therapy will depend on the instillation of trust and motivation that the therapist and the client can develop from the first contact. At this stage, it is necessary for the therapist to carefully avoid ending the session with the stabilization of the client (Zaro et al., 1980).

Kuyken et al. (2010), mention that case conceptualization can be seen as a metaphor for a cauldron, where the therapist can combine several different substances to obtain something new. In this way, the therapist will investigate the individual history of the client. Through the experiences and evidence that theory and research present, a therapist will follow a protocol based on the singular history of the individual to approach the formulation of a case. Table 3.1 is a model of anamnesis, according to the same authors.

The conceptualization of cases in CBT becomes an important map for the therapist to use in scientific intervention and to draw up an individualized treatment plan using techniques that enable the client to develop new learning and manage emotional regulation (Sauer-Zavala et al., 2017; Schweizer et al., 2020).

Clinical Case

"F", 18 years old, male, was born in Brazil and lived with his maternal grandparents since he was 3 years old. The mother, having been abandoned by her husband, moved to the United States, and left him with his grandparents. "F" claims to have no relationship with his biological father, who abandoned him.

"F's" maternal grandmother was practically his mother, and she passed away last year. Without an alternative, "F" had to come to the United States to try to build a healthier emotional life. "F" did not feel safe living with his mother, who remarried for the second time and returned to Brazil. At 15 years old, "F" had worked in the fields to help the family, when he went to his mother's house, he was mistreated, assaulted, and neglected by his mother and stepfather. The stepfather was very aggressive and dangerous, he had a gun, he was diagnosed with borderline personality disorder. "F" was afraid to be with his mother and decided to continue living with his grandparents until the grandmother's death. The grandfather was already sick with diabetes and other chronic problems, so he couldn't stay with him.

His maternal aunt and uncle, who live in the USA, decided to take care of "F", as they noticed how traumatized he was by abuse, aggressiveness, and malnourishment

Table 3.1 Conceptualization model

(1) Demographic data	Name, marital status, date of birth, religion, sex, date, occupation, and telephone number
(2) Describe your difficulties and issues	What reasons brought you to therapy?
(3) What do you want to achieve with therapy?	What do you hope to achieve or resolve through therapy?
(4) Talk about your family in detail	Details about family members: mother, father, siblings, developmentally important members
(5) Talk about the most apparent characteristics in your mother and father	Striking traits in your mother and father that draw the most attention
(6) Name or describe problems in family relationships, between you and your parents, between your siblings and you, between your parents	Family issues
(7) How much does this bother you currently?	Level of discomfort with family problems
(8) How is your life currently?	Description of the environment at home/ work, favorite activities and what you don't like
(9) Describe your education and the important points of your school education	Educational history, relevant points in your academic training
(10) Describe your professional life and the important points in your life today	Significant professional path for your current life
(11) Name the experiences that have disturbed you throughout your life	Significant events throughout your life and how much they still impact you today
(12) Describe the abuse and/or trauma you have experienced	Experiences of past abusive relationships and traumas
(13) Describe your emotional and physical health history	History of emotional and physical health, medication use, chronic illnesses, treatments
(14) History of use, abuse, or dependence on substances (alcohol or drugs)	History of substance use, abuse, or dependence
(15) What are your future plans?	Aspirations and dreams for the future

due to neglect of food by his mother and stepfather. His relatives were terrified when they saw their nephew when he arrived in the United States, very beaten down and scared of the life he had in Brazil and sad for the loss of the grandmother who was his protector.

"F" finished High School, without having another chance for a better future in his city, he agreed to come to his aunt and uncle's house in the United States. During the psychological evaluation sessions, "F" presented as anxious and downcast when telling his story. He showed some physical symptoms of anxiety, such as tachycardia, sweating, and tremors in his hands. He mentioned several times in the sessions that he felt like a burden for the family, and so he had to work so that no one would worry about him, but that there was no problem in living alone. He reported feeling very guilty and ashamed for having to live with his aunt and uncle, as he didn't want to disrupt anyone's life. Today "F" works as a carpenter and studies English. When evaluated, he obtained the following scores: 30 for anxiety (moderate to severe), 17 for depression (mild to moderate) and 16 for hopelessness (mild to moderate).

Conceptualizing the Case Described Above

First step: The therapist will describe and summarize with the client all the important factors that interfered with his behaviors, feelings, and thoughts and that are part of his life story. Psychoeducation for trauma is carried out according to the client's individual story. In this case, "F" was abandoned by his mother at 3 years old and raised by his grandparents until he was 15. When his mother returned to Brazil married to an aggressive man with a history of serious mental problems. "F" was assaulted several times, physically and emotionally. "F" was forced to work and wasn't fed properly, as his mother and stepfather considered him a slave. He lost his grandmother at 17 and was left without emotional support.

Second step: Automatic thoughts (AT)—"I don't want to cause problems for my family"; "I don't want to depend on people", "I always think I'm disrupting other people's lives"; "people don't love me."

Third step: Intermediate and central beliefs—What is the truth about these thoughts and your life story? The feeling of having been abandoned by his mother and mistreated by his mother and stepfather makes him believe that he has no value, that he is not loved by anyone. Even though he was raised by his grandparents, with love, he felt that it was work.

Fourth step: Physiological and behavioral sensations—"F" became discouraged when telling his story, showed some physical symptoms of anxiety, such as tachycardia, sweating, and tremors in his hands.

Fifth step: The results of the anxiety tests, Depression and despair have shown that "F" meets the criteria for Post-Traumatic Stress Disorder (PTSD), which are described as: A. Exposure to a traumatic event. B. Presence of intrusive symptoms associated with the traumatic event. C. Persistent avoidance of stimuli associated with the traumatic event. D. Negative changes in mood and cognition. E. Changes in reactivity and physiological response (DSM 5 309.81; ICD 10 43.1).

Evidence Based on Protocols and the Importance of the Therapeutic Relationship in CBT Intervention

CBT emerged in the late 1960s for the treatment of depression. Currently, there are structured protocols for various disorders such as: panic disorder, social phobias, simple phobias, generalized anxiety, eating disorders, mood disorders, chemical dependency, and even for personality disorders like borderline disorder. Nowadays, empirically based transdiagnostic protocols in CBT have emerged in the twenty-first century, contextualizing a more humanized and individualized model for the conduct of collaborative and therapeutic treatment.

During therapy sessions, the therapist who works with the transdiagnostic approach, after clinical conceptualization, can use techniques such as psychoeducation, mindfulness, bibliotherapy, Socratic questioning, downward arrow guided discovery, diaphragmatic breathing, exposure, reattribution, and social skills training (Barlow et al., 2011; DeOrnelasMaia et al., 2013; Pehlivanidis et al., 2006).

The aims of the unified protocol are to achieve pre-established goals at the beginning of the process, as well as learning emotional regulation management (Barlow et al., 2011; Button et al., 2012; DeOrnelasMaia et al., 2015). In CBT, it is common for the therapist to perform a functional analysis of the case, choosing to use the intervention that ensures a variety of promising results in therapy (Bandeira et al., 2006; Guilhardi, 1998; Kohlenberg & Tsai, 2001; Rosenfarb, 1992; Zaro et al., 1980).

In addition to the functional analysis of the therapeutic relationship, the components to be taken into account for the use of treatment in transdiagnostic approaches are duration, intensity, and frequency of physical sensations, level of distress, and interference of symptoms. These variables are part of the triggers for thought distortions and common beliefs in emotional disorders, and the grading of them seems to interfere with the prognosis of treatment (Barlow et al., 2011; Sauer-Zavala et al., 2017; Tolin, 2010). The cognitive-behavioral therapist, when presenting the therapy model, proposes possible tools that can be used not only in the meeting with the client, but can also be continued as homework. This will favor the client to have a continuous therapeutic process that can promote self-knowledge and, thus, learn new ways of relating to their thoughts, sensations, and behaviors (Gould et al., 1997; Hunot et al., 2007).

Skinner in 1953, revised in 2007, laid the foundations of behavioral therapy for the development of one of the essential characteristics for a satisfactory therapeutic relationship: the therapist should have empathy and be free of judgments, that is, be a non-punitive listener. This conclusion is quite clear, as those who are suffering and seek therapy probably do so because they are punished in some way in some context of their life. The therapist's unconditional acceptance allows the client to demonstrate that they can be authentic, say what they need, and not be criticized for such behavior (Lambert, 2013; Lambert et al., 2001). An important aspect of the therapeutic relationship is the bond or alliance created between client and therapist. It is observed that each client is unique and singular in the way they relate. One of the therapist's tasks is to be attentive to the clinically relevant behaviors of the relationship. Also, according Kazantis et al. (2017) attention; listening skills; empathy; positive consideration; seek customer feedback; genuineness; trust; mutual respect and, positive relational bond with the client are qualifications that the therapists can build during the therapeutic alliance, for example, pay attention to bonding signals and the client's signals, which will convey their life experiences at every moment, in the specific way they perform their roles in the psychotherapeutic context (Kotov et al., 2017; Lambert, 2013).

In therapy, both client and therapist undergo a process of change, because, above all, there is a human relationship between individuals with their potentialities, limitations, experiences, and emotions (Monteiro, 2010). Therefore, in the first sessions of therapy it is important to establish trust, safety, and confidentiality between therapist and client.

The therapeutic relationship can be predictive of an effective outcome in the process of CBT intervention. However, it is relevant that the therapist develops some fundamental skills, such as: empathetic and understanding posture, acceptance devoid of judgments, authenticity, self-confidence, flexibility, commitment, tolerance, and interest. Regarding specific therapeutic behaviors, the most functional are the neutralization of gestural behaviors, maintaining eye contact, verbalizations about thoughts and feelings, a less directive posture, and guidance based on each client's stories (Bandeira et al., 2006).

Clinically relevant behavior variables can arise in various sessions, in this aspect it is important that the therapist perceives when the client presents some behaviors related to emotional avoidance and difficulties in establishing changes. These responses can be considered resistance, and with this, the client can increase these dysfunctional behaviors if important points to be discussed in the therapy content are not used. In this way, these very different conceptions, where the changes that the therapist expects to happen and the procedures to produce them may not coincide with those expected by the client.

Furthermore, the means by which he/she chose to achieve them may differ from original expectations. The difficulty in accepting changes and also in understanding that there is a resistance that can hinder this therapeutic evolution is a factor that if processed and included in the treatment will produce more significant effects. Moreover, if the behaviors/problems and improvements happen during the session, the propagation of this evolution makes the therapy work more effective (Guilhardi, 1998).

Kohlenberg and Tsai (1991), point out that therapists, when identifying the functional and dysfunctional aspects that maintain the problematic behaviors brought as complaints, will provide the client with a significant role in the therapeutic relationship, which will favor the collaborative participation in their development and in search of their goals.

The Therapeutic Alliance

The therapeutic alliance is defined as the collaborative aspects of the relationship that occur between the therapist-client (Flückiger et al., 2019). It is considered an essential part of all psychotherapies. It is a core competence, and one of the first and most important, to be developed by therapists. Starting from the first contact and evolving and changing during the entire therapeutic process. Whether positive or negative, the contact will directly influence the therapeutic alliance (Sperry & Sperry, 2020). As research and clinical experience highlight, the therapeutic relationship is as responsible as specific treatment methods in terms of efficacy (Norcross & Lambert, 2019).

The topic of the therapeutic relationship has been studied since the work of Sigmund Freud, who observed the need for collaboration between the therapist and client (Dobson, 2022; Lavender, 2018). Freud based himself on the transfer in relationships, and later, speculated about the collaborative aspect between therapist and client (Flückiger et al., 2019).

Also important is the work of Bordin (1979) who considered that the collaborative alliance was related to three aspects or characteristics: the emotional bond between the therapist and client, agreement on the tasks that are part of therapy, and agreeing with the treatment objectives.

As observed by Lavender (2018), CBT involves tasks, which are worked collaboratively with clients, and there are agreements on therapeutic goals. And finally, despite not seeing the bond as central in CBT, it recalls that clients need to feel understood and respected in the relationship. This is also affirmed by Kazantis et al. (2017), recognizing the need for clients to feel respected, understood, valued, and comfortable, to promote the sharing of their personal experiences.

In a humanistic line, Rogers (1957) pointed out necessary conditions for therapeutic change, such as empathic understanding and unconditional positive regard. The warm encounter of two people was considered more effective in the change process than the set of techniques. Empathy, unconditional acceptance, and collaboration between therapist and client contribute to the creation of a safe and encouraging environment (Beck, 2021). CBT brings a bit of the Rogerian influence, with respect to what are called generic elements of the alliance. Kazantis and Dobson (2022) emphasize that empathic understanding, plus effective interpersonal style, are central points with respect to evaluations of therapist skills.

In CBT, the authors recognize the therapist-client relationship as a predictive factor for a better therapeutic outcome (Beck, 2021; Dobson & Dobson, 2018; Gilbert & Leahy, 2007; Lavender, 2018). Since the beginning of CBT, studies by Aaron Beck et al. (1979) dedicated themselves to talking about the therapeutic relationship, highlighting skills of accuracy, empathy, authenticity, basic trust, and rapport. As Beck (2021) points out, if the therapist cannot express these competencies, there will be a need for supervision or training, with the aim of improving them. The therapeutic relationship has been perceived since the publication of Aaron Beck et al. (1979) and more recently, as necessary, although not sufficient for change (Cornacchio et al., 2017; Kazantis & Dobson, 2022).

The therapeutic relationship includes generic elements: empathy, expression of positive regard, and also specific elements of CBT: collaborative empiricism and Socratic dialogue, which directly facilitate various mechanisms of change, such as cognitive reappraisal, acceptance, identification of emotions, and coping (Kazantis & Dobson, 2022).

Positive relational bond with the client with these generic elements can facilitate the process and demonstrate the importance of valuing the client and encouraging him to engage in tasks. The therapist through empathy can provide support and understand the client, in such a way that he can explore alternative thoughts and ideas (Moorey & Lavender, 2018). The same authors recognize the need for empathy, so that the therapist can validate the individual, and show the client that he is understood during the therapeutic process.

Collaborative empiricism, also called empirical collaboration, refers to teamwork (Dobson & Dobson, 2018; Kazantis et al., 2017), where the client and the therapist work together to identify the problems, make decisions, formulate hypotheses, and test them, as well as requesting client feedback, so that the therapeutic process is a shared responsibility with the aim of effecting change.

The collaborative therapeutic style seeks suggestions, opinions, and ideas from clients about their priorities (Kazantis et al., 2017). Thus, it allows for the adjustment of tasks that occur between sessions, as evidence emerges about which changes are most adaptive for the client (Dobson, 2022).

Empiricism is characterized by the therapist helping the client to adopt the scientific method in light of their experiences, in order to verify, test their thoughts, understand beliefs, and consider adaptive alternatives (Kazantis et al., 2017).

Socratic dialogue involves empirical collaboration, presenting itself as a strategy for changing cognitions (Kazantis & Dobson, 2022). It is considered a respectful style in the interaction between the therapist and the client, in a posture of learning to understand the client through inductive questions and reflective dialogue, with the ultimate goal of understanding the problems, and suggesting other paths (Dobson & Dobson, 2018). Socratic dialogue promotes the active involvement of the client, whose questions are supportive and respectful, considering the client's knowledge, and focused on what is being discussed, involving genuine curiosity and the client's experience (Kazantis et al., 2017).

Adapting the Relationship

Beck (2021) and Kazantis et al. (2017), agree that an essential aspect is the ability for a therapist to adapt. Adaptation of skills, techniques, and approach are crucial considering that each client is specific. Since each client is unique, each therapeutic relationship becomes unique. Some clients may welcome empathy, while others may feel uncomfortable or suspicious. Therefore, emotional reactions during the session should be considered.

Understanding cultures and other characteristics, such as age, gender, ethnicity, socioeconomic level, and sexual orientation are critical. The fact is that the therapeutic relationship requires adaptation and variation for each client. Adaptations are based on the evolution of cognitive conceptualization of cases, aiming at the involvement of clients with the techniques used, which must exist within the context of the relationship (Kazantis & Dobson, 2022).

As Beck (2021) rightly observed, each client is an individual, for whom a conceptualization and individualized treatment plan is developed. From the point of view of an age factor, the child population is usually referred by their parents, schools, or other services, to treat problems that the client often believes they do not have. It is necessary to adapt the relationship, incorporating games, play therapy, understanding family variables, among them values, preferences, culture, and school influences (Cornacchio et al., 2017).

According to Feindler and Smerling (2022) the alliance in child treatment is certainly more complex than in adult therapy, considering multiple alliances to be attended to. They involve the parents who made the decision to start, continue, or end therapy. Likewise, their cooperation is essential so that the children can complete their tasks. Therefore, a good alliance with the child, parents, or caregivers is necessary.

The Therapist

The therapeutic relationship cannot be treated only from the point of view of the clients' thoughts and beliefs. The role of the therapist in the therapeutic relationship also needs to be observed, highlighting their interpersonal side. They have their own processes and are also human beings who struggle with their own problems. It is necessary for the therapist to pay attention to their own thoughts, conceptualize their own relational history, such as their own beliefs, have a respectful attitude towards clients, while seeking continuous self-growth (Kazantis et al., 2017). Situations in therapy can trigger thoughts, feelings, and behaviors that can be problematic. The therapist may perceive themselves as a terrible therapist, presenting feelings of frustration and guilt.

CBT itself does not bring the concept of countertransference, as addressed in psychodynamic therapy, although Gilbert and Leahy (2007) and Leahy (2003), in their texts address the issue, it is worth noting that certain clients and their behaviors can trigger reactions in the therapist. Self-case conceptualization is encouraged, allowing one to see their own core beliefs and values. Self-reflective exercises have been useful in understanding the processes that occur in therapeutic interactions (Bennett-Levy et al., 2001). Self-practice and self-reflection are encouraged so that one can understand their own stories, their schemas and beliefs, and their own vulnerabilities (Kazantis et al., 2017). They are also encouraged to record thoughts about themselves, which are useful in difficult relationship situations, or to understand some processes that occur in the session.

Self-practice can enhance learning, as well as the development of the CBT therapist. Self-reflection allows one to reflect on their own experience, generating questions about how they have been providing services to clients. Self-reflection allows for distancing and reflection on one's own experiences and cognitive, emotional, and behavioral patterns as a professional (Bennett-Levy et al., 2001). It allows one to understand oneself and recognize how their thoughts and emotions are triggered in the therapeutic process (Bennett-Levy & Haarhoff, 2019).

It is worth remembering that to stay active in the therapy process with promising results, the therapist needs certain support, such as continuing education and clinical supervision. Supervision, for example, is an opportunity for knowledge acquisition and maintenance of therapeutic skills, but also for modeling an interpersonal style. Feedback in supervision may not be a rewarding experience, in fact, it can be sometimes stressful. Though feedback is not always positive, it is part of the process of life as a whole, especially for the therapist who is dedicated to their client's improvement and growth (Kazantis et al., 2017).

Conclusion

In CBT, case conceptualization involves understanding a client's problems. Given a detailed formulation that the therapist builds by synthesizing the gathered information, identifying core beliefs and patterns, and planning target interventions to address the client's specific challenges as a roadmap for effective treatment in CBT. For that it is relevant that therapist and client can build a therapeutic alliance which emphasizes a strong, collaborative relationship between the therapist and client to enhance treatment effectiveness.

References

Aldao, A., & Nolen-Hoeksema, S. (2010). Specificity of cognitive emotion regulation strategies: A transdiagnostic examination. *Behaviour Research and Therapy, 48*(10), 974–983. https://doi.org/10.1016/j.brat.2010.06.002. Epub 2010 Jun 12. PMID: 20591413.

Andrade, L. H., Wang, Y. P., Andreoni, S., Silveira, C. M., Alexandrino-Silva, C., Siu, E. R., Nishimura, R., Anthony, J. C., Gattaz, W. F., Kessler, R. C., & Viana, M. C. (2012). Mental disorders in megacities: Findings from the São Paulo megacity mental health survey, Brazil. *PLoS One, 7*(2), e31879. https://doi.org/10.1371/journal.pone.0031879. Epub 2012 Feb 14. PMID: 22348135; PMCID: PMC3279422.

Bandeira, M., Quaglia, M. A. C., Freitas, L. C., de Sousa, A. M., Costa, A. L. P., Gomides, M. M. P., & Lima, P. B. (2006). Habilidades interpessoais na atuação do psicólogo. *Interação, 10*(1), 139–149. https://doi.org/10.15689/ap.2020.1903.15832.02

Barlow, D. H., Farchione, T. J., Firholme, C. P., Ellard, K. K., Boisseau, C. L., Allen, L. B., & Ehrenreich-May, J. (2011). *Unified protocol for transdiagnostic treatment of emotional disorders. Therapist guide.ThatWork.* Oxford University Press.

Beck, J. S. (2021). *Cognitive behavior therapy: Basics and beyond* (3rd ed.). The Guilford Press.

Beck, A. T., Rush, A., Shaw, B., & Emery, G. (1979). *Cognitive therapy of depression.* The Guilford Press.

Bennett-Levy, J., & Haarhoff, B. (2019). Why therapists need to take a good look at themselves: Self-practice/self-reflection as an integrative training strategy for evidence-based practices. In S. Dimidjian (Ed.), *Evidence-based practice in action: Bridging clinical science and intervention* (pp. 380–394). The Guilford Press.

Bennett-Levy, J., Turner, F., Beaty, T., Smith, M., Paterson, B., & Farmer, S. (2001). The value of self-practice of cognitive therapy techniques and self-reflection in the training of cognitive therapists. *Behavioural and Cognitive Psychotherapy, 29*(2), 203–220. https://doi.org/10.1017/S1352465801002077

Bordin, E. S. (1979). The generalizability of the psychoanalytic concept of the working alliance. *Psychotherapy: Theory, Research & Practice, 16*(3), 252–260. https://doi.org/10.1037/h0085885

Brown, T. A., & Barlow, D. H. (2002). Classification of anxiety and mood disorders. In D. H. Barlow (Ed.), *Anxiety and its disorders: The nature and treatment of anxiety and panic* (2nd ed., pp. 292–327). The Guilford Press.

Button, K. S., Wiles, N. J., Lewis, G., Peters, T. J., & Kessler, D. (2012). Factors associated with differential response to online cognitive behavioural therapy. *Social Psychiatry and Psychiatric Epidemiology, 47*(5), 827–833. https://doi.org/10.1007/s00127-011-0389-1. Epub 2011 May 4. PMID: 21541696.

Cape, J., Whittington, C., Buszewicz, M., Wallace, P., & Underwood, L. (2010). Brief psychological therapies for anxiety and depression in primary care: Meta-analysis and meta-regression. *BMC Medicine, 25*, 8–38. https://doi.org/10.1186/1741-7015-8-38. PMID: 20579335; PMCID: PMC2908553.

Cornacchio, D., Sanchez, A., Chou, T., & Comer, J. (2017). Cognitive-behavioral therapy for children and adolescents. In S. Hofmann & G. Asmundson (Eds.), *The science of cognitive behavioral therapy*. Academic.

Craddock, N., & Owen, M. J. (2010). The Kraepelinian dichotomy—Going, going...but still not gone. *The British Journal of Psychiatry, 196*, 92–95. https://doi.org/10.1192/bjp.bp.109.073429. PMID: 20118450; PMCID: PMC2815936.

DeOrnelasMaia, A. C. C., Braga, A. A., Nunes, C. A., Nardi, A. E., & Silva, A. C. (2013). Transdiagnostic treatment using a unified protocol: Application for patients with a range of comorbid mood and anxiety disorders. *Trends Psychiatry Psychother [online], 35*(2), 134–140. https://doi.org/10.1590/s2237-60892013000200007. PMID: 25923304.

DeOrnelasMaia, A. C. C., Nardi, A. E., & Cardoso, A. (2015). The utilization of unified protocols in behavioral cognitive therapy in transdiagnostic group subjects: A clinical trial. *Journal of Affective Disorders, 172*, 179–183. https://doi.org/10.1016/j.jad.2014.09.023. Epub 2014 Sep 28. PMID: 25451415.

Dobson, K. (2022). Therapeutic relationship. *Cognitive and Behavioral Practice, 29*, 51–544. https://doi.org/10.1016/j.cbpra.2022.02.006

Dobson, D., & Dobson, K. (2018). *Evidence-based practice of cognitive-behavioral therapy* (2nd ed.). The Guilford Press.

Feindler, E. L., & Smerling, C. (2022). A review of therapeutic alliance and child CBT. *Child & Family Behavior Therapy, 44*(1), 18–34. https://doi.org/10.1080/07317107.2022.2027191

Flückiger, C., Del Re, A. C., Wampold, B., & Horvath. (2019). Alliance in adult psychotherapy. In J. Norcross & M. Lambert (Eds.), *Psychotherapy relationships that work. Volume: 1 evidence-based therapist contributions* (3rd ed.). Oxford University Press.

Gilbert, P., & Leahy, R. L. (Eds.). (2007). *The therapeutic relationship in the cognitive behavioral psychotherapies*. Routledge/Taylor & Francis Group.

Gould, R. A., Otto, M. W., Pollack, M. H., & Yap, L. (1997). Cognitive behavioral and pharmacological treatment of generalized anxiety disorder: A preliminary meta-analyis. *Behavior Therapy, 28*(2), 285–305. https://doi.org/10.1016/S0005-7894(97)80048-2

Guilhardi, H. J. (1998). *A Resistência do Cliente à Mudanças*. Parte deste trabalho foi apresentado numa mesa redonda no I Congresso de Psicoterapias Cognitivas Latino-Americanas e I Congresso Brasileiro de Psicoterapias Cognitivas, realizados de 2 a 4 de abril de 1998 em Gramado (RS). http://www.terapiaporcontingencias.com.br/. Acesso em: 03/12/2023.

Hunot, V., Churchill, R., Silva, L. M., & Teixeira, V. (2007). Psychological therapies for generalized anxiety disorder. *Cochrane Database of Systematic Reviews, 24*(1), CD001848. https://doi.org/10.1002/14651858.CD001848.pub4. PMID: 17253466; PMCID: PMC7025441.

Johansson, R., Sjöberg, E., Sjögren, M., Johnsson, E., Carlbring, P., Andersson, T., Rousseau, A., Andersson, G., & Tailored, V. S. (2012). Standardized internet-based cognitive behavior therapy for depression and comorbid symptoms: A randomized controlled trial. *PLoS One, 7*(5), e36905. https://doi.org/10.1371/journal.pone.0036905. Epub 2012 May 15. PMID: 22615841; PMCID: PMC3352859.

Johnston, L., Titov, N., Andrews, G., Spence, J., & Dear, B. F. (2011). A RCT of a transdiagnostic internet-delivered treatment for three anxiety disorders: Examination of support roles and disorder-specific outcomes. *PLoS One, 6*(11), e28079. https://doi.org/10.1371/journal.pone.0028079

Kazantis, N., & Dobson, K. (2022). Therapeutic relationships in cognitive behavioral therapy: Theory and recent research. *Special Section: Part 1: Psychotherapy Relationships in Cognitive Behavioral Therapy, 32*(8). https://doi.org/10.1080/10503307.2022.2124047. Epub 2022 Oct 6. PMID: 36201793.

Kazantis, N., Dattilio, F., & Dobson, K. (2017). *The therapeutic relationship in cognitive-behavioral therapy: A clinician's guide*. Guilford Publications.

Kohlenberg, R. J., & Tsai, M. (1991). Functional analytic psychotherapy: Creating intense and curative therapeutic relationships. *Plenum Press*. https://doi.org/10.1007/978-0-387-70855-3

Kohlenberg, R., & Tsai, M. (2001). *Psicoterapia Analítica Funcional*. ESETec. Editores Associados. https://doi.org/10.1037/h0100941

Kotov, R., Krueger, R. F., Watson, D., Achenbach, T. M., Althoff, R. R., Bagby, R. M., & Zimmerman, M. (2017). The Hierarchical Taxonomy of Psychopathology (HITOP): A dimensional alternative to traditional nosologies. *Journal of Abnormal Psychology, 126*, 454–477. https://doi.org/10.1037/abn0000258. Epub 2017 Mar 23. PMID: 28333488.

Kraus, D. R., Castonguay, L., Boswell, J. F., Nordberg, S. S., & Hayes, J. A. (2011). Therapist effectiveness: Implications for accountability and patient care. *Psychotherapy Research, 21*(3), 267–276. https://doi.org/10.1080/10503307.2011.563249

Kuyken, W., Padesky, C., & Dudley, R. (2010). *Conceituação de casos colaborativos: o trabalho em equipe com pacientes em terapia cognitivo-comportamental*. Artmed.

Lambert, M. J. (2013). Outcome in psychotherapy: The past and important advances. *Psychotherapy (Chicago, Ill.), 50*(1), 42–51. https://doi.org/10.1037/a0030682. PMID: 23505980.

Lambert, M. J., Whipple, J. L., Smart, D.W., Vermeersch, D. A., Nielsen, S. L., Hawkins E. J. (2001). *The effects of providing therapists with feedback on client progress during psychotherapy: are outcomes enhanced? Psychother Res, 11*, 49–68.

Lavender, A. (2018). The therapeutic alliance building a collaborative relationship and managing challenges. In S. Moorey & A. Lavender (Eds.), *The therapeutic relationship in cognitive behavioral therapy*. Sage.

Leahy, R. (2003). *Overcoming resistance in cognitive therapy*. The Guilford Publications.

Marçal, J. V. (2005). Estabelecendo Objetivos na Prática Clínica: Quais Caminhos Seguir? *Revista Brasileira de Terapia Comportamental e Cognitiva, VII*(2), 231–245. Recuperado em 03 de dezembro de 2023, de http://pepsic.bvsalud.org/scielo.php?script=sci_arttext&pid=S1517-55452005000200008&lng=pt&tlng=pt

Monteiro, M. (2010). *Do apego ao cuidado: Implicações do Vínculo Afetivo na Perspectiva Clínica*. http://www.redepsi.com.br/portal/modules/smartsection/item.php?itemid=1664. Recuperado em 03 de dezembro de 2023, de http://pepsic.bvsalud.org/scielo.php?script=sci_arttext&pid=S1809-52672005000100003&lng=pt&tlng=pt

Moorey, S., & Lavender, A. (2018). *The therapeutic relationship in cognitive behavioral therapy*. Sage.

Norcross, J., & Lambert, M. (2019). Psychotherapy relationships that work. In *Volume: 1 evidence-based therapist contributions* (3rd ed.). Oxford University Press. https://doi.org/10.1093/med-psych/9780190843953.003.0001

Pehlivanidis, A., Papanikolaou, K., Politis, A., Liossi, A., Daskalopoulou, E., Gournellis, R., Soldatos, M., Papakosta, V. M., Zervas, I., & Papakostas, Y. G. (2006). The screening role of an introductory course in cognitive therapy training. *Academic Psychiatry, 30*(3), 196–199. https://doi.org/10.1176/appi.ap.30.3.196

Rogers, C. R. (1957). The necessary and sufficient conditions of therapeutic personality change. *Journal of Consulting Psychology, 21*, 95–103. https://doi.org/10.1037/h0045357

Rosenfarb, I. S. (1992). *Uma Interpretação Analítica Comportamental da Relação Terapêutica*. The Psychological Record. Tradução: Profª Lydia Akemy Onesti.

Ruggero, C. J., Kotov, R., Hopwood, C. J., First, M., Clark, L. A., Skodol, A. E., et al. (2019). Integrating the Hierarchical Taxonomy of Psychopathology (HiTOP) into clinical practice. *Journal of Consulting and Clinical Psychology, 87*, 1069–1084. https://doi.org/10.1037/ccp0000452. PMID: 31724426; PMCID: PMC6859953.

Sauer-Zavala, S., Gutner, C. A., Farchione, T. J., Boettcher, H. T., Bullis, J. R., & Barlow, D. H. (2017). Current definitions of "transdiagnostic" in treatment development: A search for consensus. *Behavior Therapy, 48*, 128–138. https://doi.org/10.1016/j.beth.2016.09.004

Schweizer, T. H., Snyder, H. R., Young, J. F., & Hankin, B. L. (2020). The breadth and potency of transdiagnostic cognitive risks for psycho-pathology in youth. *Journal of Consulting and Clinical Psychology, 88*, 196–211. https://doi.org/10.1037/ccp0000470

Skinner, B. F. (2007). *Ciência e Comportamento Humano* (J. C. Todorov, & R. Azzi, Trads.,11ª ed.). Martins fontes. (Obra original publicada em 1953)

Sperry, L., & Sperry, J. (2020). *Case conceptualization. Mastering this competency with ease and confidence* (2nd ed.). Routledge. https://doi.org/10.4324/9780429288968

Steele, S. J., Farchione, T. J., Cassiello-Robbins, C., Ametaj, A., Sbi, S., Sauer-Zavala, S., & Barlow, D. H. (2018). Efficacy of the unified protocol for transdiagnostic treatment of comorbid psychopathology accompanying emotional disorders compared to treatments targeting single disorders. *Journal of Psychiatric Research, 104*, 211–216. https://doi.org/10.1016/j.jpsychires.2018.08.005. PMID: 30103069; PMCID: PMC6219859.

Tolin, D. F. (2010). Is cognitive-behavioral therapy more effective than other therapies? A meta-analytic review. *Clinical Psychology Review, 30*(6), 710–720. https://doi.org/10.1016/j.cpr.2010.05.003. Epub 2010 May 25. PMID: 20547435.

Zaro, J. S., Barach, R., & Nedelman, D. J. (1980). *Algumas Habilidades Terapêuticas mais Refinadas. Introdução à Prática Psicoterapêutica*. EPO.

Zitman, F. G. (2012). ROM in mood, anxiety and somatoform disorders: A promising technique with pleasing results. *Tijdschr Psychiatr, 54*(2), 173–177. Dutch. PMID: 22331540.

Chapter 4
Contributions of Functional Analytic Psychotherapy for the Development of More Transdiagnostic Interventions in Cognitive Behavioral Therapies

Pricila Albrecht Bornholdt and Camilla Volpato Broering

Introduction

In the past, CBT (Cognitive Behavioral Therapy) sessions were structured based on the severity of mental disorders, and the intervention was focused on changing problematic behavior. Over the years, a new model emerged based on the emotional processes of transdiagnostic patients. This new concept originates from the identification of common processes characterized across various diagnoses or even in the absence of a diagnosis. The client will bring various complaints or issues to the office that are not related to a single disorder. In the transdiagnostic perspective, what matters most is the intensity, frequency, and durability of emotions, and with that, the potential for developing models and interventions focused on these processes.

As a result, there has been a significant increase in research aimed at understanding change processes in CBT and a decrease in research focused on evaluating specific protocols for specific disorders (Sauer-Zavala et al., 2017). In this scenario, the development of transdiagnostic treatments began. The objective of these treatment models is to understand the common cognitive, emotional, and behavioral factors across different psychiatric disorders that contribute to the development of psychopathology and psychological distress. These factors are referred to as risk factors, maladaptive or dysfunctional coping strategies, or simply transdiagnostic factors (Leahy, 2002; McKay et al., 2011).

Research in transdiagnostic treatments has shown that, in reality, the way one responds to stress and emotions assessed as negative through the chosen strategies

P. A. Bornholdt (✉)
Mondaí, SC, Brazil

C. V. Broering
Universidade do Vale do Itajaí (UNIVALI), Itajaí, SC, Brazil

A. C. Ornelas (ed.), *Transdiagnostic Approaches in Cognitive Behavioral Therapy*, https://doi.org/10.1007/978-3-031-63494-9_4

will largely determine the emergence or absence of emotional problems (Hayes & Hoffman, 2018). In contrast to standardized protocols that follow a specific order of intervention, in transdiagnostic treatment, the intervention is directed and adapted based on the dysfunctional coping strategies most commonly used by the client in reality. Therefore, it should be discussed with the client how emotional states affect our cognitions, physiological responses, and behaviors, how emotions can be understood, and how issues related to emotions arise.

According to Hayes and Hoffman (2018), the objective would be to understand the core biopsychosocial processes that should be targeted with a specific client, identify the patient's goals in a particular situation, and then determine the component methods that are most likely to modify these processes. The identification of core processes in psychotherapy will guide the therapist and help avoid the limitations of treatment protocols based on a rigid and arbitrary system, directly linking the treatment to theory. This perspective will guide this chapter, aiming to consolidate many existing trends and build on the strengths of the various generations of work that make up the approaches of Cognitive and Behavioral Therapies.

Various transdiagnostic interventions have been observed to develop, such as Acceptance and Commitment Therapy (ACT) with its model of psychopathology anchored in psychological inflexibility, Dialectical Behavioral Therapy (DBT) with its focus on emotional dysregulation issues, and Functional Analytic Psychotherapy (FAP) which emphasizes the role of the therapeutic relationship as a promoter of clinical improvements. This chapter's goal is to write about the latter.

Fundamental Aspects of FAP

Functional Analytic Psychotherapy (FAP) is a third-generation/wave therapy within Cognitive and Behavioral Therapies, based on the epistemological assumptions of Radical Behaviorism. Through empirically established analytical behavioral processes such as learning, reinforcement, and modeling, FAP uses the therapeutic relationship as the primary tool to enhance the client's interpersonal and intimacy repertoires. FAP believes that the therapeutic relationship shares functional similarities with other relationships the client establishes in their daily life. Therefore, it is understood that behaviors causing harm to the client's life will also occur in the therapy session. This is a significant premise for determining whether a problem is suitable for FAP treatment (Kohlenberg & Tsai, 1991).

The client's behaviors that are the subject of their complaints and that occur during the therapy session are referred to as Clinically Relevant Behaviors of Type 1—CRB1. It is common at the beginning of treatment for these behaviors to occur frequently during the session. On the other hand, Clinically Relevant Behaviors of Type 2—CRB2 are the client's improvement behaviors during the session. These are the therapeutic targets defined functionally and idiosyncratically, and they are expected to occur progressively as therapy progresses. Clinically Relevant Behaviors of Type 3—CRB3 are classified as such when the client establishes a functional interpretation of their behaviors during the session. Identifying the different CRBs occurring in the session is considered by Tsai et al. (2009a) to be the heart of FAP, as therapeutic goals are established through this identification.

For FAP, the mechanism that enables client change/improvement is anchored through genuine and social reinforcement provided by the therapist during the session, contingent on the client's CRB2s. Therefore, the authors suggest five rules to guide the therapist's behavior in achieving therapeutic goals. Rule 1 advises the therapist to be attentive to the CRBs occurring during the session. Rule 2 encourages the therapist to evoke CRBs so that, through Rule 3, the therapist can genuinely reinforce the presented CRB2. In Rule 4, the therapist is directed to assess the impact of the therapist's response (potential reinforcement) on the client. Rule 5 instructs the therapist to assist the client in interpreting the interaction and their CRBs during the session to promote the generalization of the learned repertoire to the client's everyday life (Tsai et al., 2009a).

A key point emphasized by Hartmann et al. (2018) highlights the importance of differentiating the **interpersonal process** occurring in the therapy session from the **content** of the client's speech, characterized by the topic the client is discussing. The interpersonal process refers to how the client, throughout the session, develops and has their repertoire modified by the therapist. In other words, it concerns the interaction between both (client and therapist) occurring in the present moment, which enables the main mechanism of change in FAP. According to these authors, this differentiation is essential because, from the perspective of FAP, the goal is to establish functional similarities between what happens in the client's everyday life and what they present in the session. In this context, understood as a safer space, the client can take risks and behave differently from what they are accustomed to in other relationships. Thus, after strengthening this repertoire in the session, the client is encouraged to act differently in other contexts outside the therapy room, in order to implement these changes in their life.

By establishing the therapeutic relationship as the social microcosm (Tsai et al., 2009b) from which the case formulation is developed and as a primary tool for conducting necessary interventions, it is essential in FAP to consider the therapist's person in this process. Evaluating each case includes weighing the therapist's characteristics that may hinder or facilitate therapeutic progress. Factors such as the therapist's life history, working style, as well as their interpersonal skills repertoire can have these effects. It is a crucial role of the therapist to develop awareness of these potential impacts in order to manage them skillfully and carefully in their interactions with clients. From this perspective, therapist behaviors that may hinder progress in the session are classified as T1, and behaviors that support the client's improvement are referred to as T2. It's important to note that just as there is no predefined definition of the client's CRBs, the therapist's Ts are not established in advance either. They should be functionally defined based on each individual case.

However, for tracking and increasing awareness of their Ts, Tsai et al. (2009a) suggest that therapists reflect on certain questions about their clients, listed below. These questions include: "What do you tend to avoid addressing with your clients? How does this avoidance impact the work that you do with these clients? What do you tend to avoid dealing with in your life? (e.g., tasks, people, memories, needs, feelings)? How do your daily life avoidances impact the work that you do with your clients?" (p. 92). According to the authors, it is crucial for the therapist to invest in their personal development, which is also an ethical consideration, as it is recommended that they assess their own reactions to the client as part of the case formulation. Otherwise, it is unlikely that the therapist can distinguish the client's CRBs occurring in the session. For example, if a client feels invalidated by something the therapist said and becomes upset and changes the subject, if the therapist has difficulty dealing with conflicts and negative feedback (potential T1), they will most likely have difficulty noticing the client's withdrawal (potential CRB1) and also promoting an honest and open discussion (T2) about the interaction that could evoke a CRB2 in the client.

Practicing FAP, as outlined by Kanter et al. (2010), demands sensitivity to the nuances that occur in the interaction between the therapist and the client. In this regard, the therapist is required to have the ability to hold intense emotions during the session. Simultaneously, they need to navigate this interaction while mapping their own emotions and understanding the case formulation and what is necessary to achieve the therapeutic goals for that client.

Given the complexity and emotional intensity of this task, Tsai et al. (2019) emphasize the importance of making the therapeutic relationship an interaction that conveys, through the therapist's attitudes, a sense of safety, trust, rapport, authenticity, and openness to vulnerability on the part of both the therapist and the client, all in the interest of the client's growth. Therefore, it is of utmost importance that, at the beginning of treatment, the therapist explicitly explains the premises of FAP to the client, with the aim of obtaining the client's verbal consent, as many seek therapy without knowing about the intense therapeutic relationship that arises in FAP.

The Importance of Social Connection in FAP

The pragmatic and functional perspective of Radical Behaviorism provided the foundation upon which FAP was created. Throughout its development, FAP integrated the principles of Contextual Behavioral Science (CBS), emphasizing the historical and current context of learning and behavior emission, while also incorporating important insights from the Science of Social Connection. FAP places significant importance on understanding the impacts that the social context can have on individuals, both in terms of their psychological functioning and their interactions and overall well-being (Holman et al., 2017).

The findings from the Science of Social Connection reveal scientifically robust studies where factors such as loneliness, social isolation, low integration, and perception of social support, as well as poor or limited relationships in terms of intimacy, increase the risk of mortality as much as excessive smoking, obesity, or continuous exposure to pollution. The assessment of these data allows us to assert that quality relationships are strong protective factors, not only at a psychological level but holistically for the individual. These variables are highlighted as fundamental for health, longevity, and happiness (Holt-Lunstad et al., 2010).

As Holman et al. (2017) point out, psychological difficulties and/or psychiatric disorders are significantly linked to a stressful social context that influences individuals' functioning, causing psychological stressors that, in turn, amplify social stress. Understanding this interconnection, and especially how improved social interaction can lead to improvement on various levels for individuals, holds a prominent place for FAP. Here again, the therapeutic relationship plays a crucial role in providing both opportunity and responsibility, considering that it can greatly influence the reinforcement of healthier behaviors and reduce harm to individuals.

The Intimacy Model in FAP

In understanding that a lack of social connections and quality intimate relationships correlates with the development of psychological disorders, it is essential to establish the concept of intimacy and healthy relationships from the perspective of FAP. To do this, the primary authors (Tsai et al., 2009b) adopted the behavioral definition of intimacy operationalized by Cordova and Scott (2001), describing a process in which an individual first emits a behavior potentially vulnerable to interpersonal punishment, and subsequently, another individual responds to this vulnerable behavior in a way that reinforces this response. Vulnerable behavior is defined as one that has been punished in the life history of that individual. In other words, there is a risk involved in emitting this behavior, and when it is reinforced instead of punished, an intimate relationship is established.

Holman et al. (2017) note that there is a key pattern that occurs repeatedly in healthy intimate relationships, precisely as described above. This process is widely prevalent in social interactions and also occurs in psychotherapy, as clients open up to vulnerability that may have been punished in another context, and the therapist responds with validation to reinforce the client's courageous behavior. In Maitland et al. (2017), a model of intimacy for FAP is proposed and detailed, consistent with the interpersonal process model of intimacy (Reis & Patrick, 1996; Reis & Shaver, 1988). This model describes the vulnerability-responsiveness relations (VRRs) process, which is empirically established as fundamental to intimate relationships.

The VRRs are characterized as a process in which intimacy is established through a dyadic interaction involving a speaker and a listener. In this interaction, the speaker presents vulnerability evoked by their context, and the listener responds with understanding and acceptance, expressing security to the speaker. The listener's response is theoretically characterized as a natural reinforcement, increasing the chances of the speaker subsequently expressing vulnerability and further fostering the experience of intimacy in this dyad (Cordova & Scott, 2001). This construct is supported and observed, as noted by Holman et al. (2017), in a broad spectrum of relationships, consistent with transdisciplinary findings (Reis, 2007). This strengthens its assumption in the FAP Intimacy Model, named The Awareness, Courage, and Love Model (ACL Model).

The ACL Model (Maitland et al., 2017) proposes that both the speaker and the listener's responses are guided by antecedents characterized as a set of skills necessary to discriminate relevant events in the context (both intrapersonal and interpersonal), which can indicate the opportunity for courageous and/or responsive responses. In this sense, these relevant events can be private, involving intrapersonal aspects such as awareness of one's needs, values, sensations, feelings, and thoughts (termed as self-awareness in the model). They can also be public, indicating experiences in interpersonal interaction, through the recognition of needs and their potential impact on the other person (termed as other-awareness in the model).

The model then unfolds into three sub-relations, in each of which the expected behavior of the speaker and the listener is specified to foster intimacy in the dyad. In the first sub-relation, it is expected that the speaker expresses emotions, while the listener's response would be to express security and acceptance. In the second sub-relation, the speaker is required to appropriately engage in emotional self-disclosure aligned with what is requested, while the listener should skillfully respond with validation. The third sub-relation specifies that the speaker should skillfully ask for something they need, while the listener's role is to provide what is requested or, if not possible, express understanding and validation in response to the request made.

The analysis and case formulation in FAP from the perspective of these sub-relations allow for the identification of behavioral excesses and/or deficits that may compromise the development of an intimacy process as described. Thus, the authors suggest using the ACL Model in a case formulation within the FAP perspective, in conjunction with the identification of CRBs (Maitland et al., 2017). The ACL model is also consistent with the initial presentation of these terms in Tsai et al. (2009a), where they are correlated with FAP rules. The term "courage" is attributed to a class of behaviors understood as vulnerable (Rule 2) and presented by the speaker, while the term "love" (Rule 3) is used to name a class of responsive behaviors from the listener in response to the speaker. To skillfully respond to these classes, it is necessary for the speaker and listener to be under the control of the terms named as self-awareness and other-awareness (Rule 1), described as the behavioral ability to recognize important private events from other antecedents in order to enhance interaction in the dyad.

For instance, when making a request (third sub-relation), it's important for the speaker to identify their needs (involving self-awareness) and to some extent anticipate the impact of this request on the listener (involving other-awareness). In summary, this model articulates a set of behaviors denoted by the term awareness, courage, and love, defined from middle-level terms, aiming to be a tool that facilitates the definition of clinical targets in the assessment process in FAP.

In addition to the ACL Model, the Functional and Ideographic Assessment System (FIAT) developed by Callaghan (2006) is a robust proposal that describes and breaks down into five functional classes important aspects in interaction with others that impact the development and maintenance of healthy intimate relationships. These are: assertion of needs, bidirectional communication, conflict, self-disclosure and intimacy, and expression and emotional experience. Both models, ACL and FIAT, are listed as useful tools for assessment in FAP. However, as proposed by Holman et al. (2017), "Given all of the existing evidence, including our own experience, if your client's presenting problem involves difficulty with intimacy, we venture that ACL may be worth assessing," p. 69.

FAP and Its Essentially Transdiagnostic Characteristic

According to Holman et al. (2017), FAP is a transdiagnostic approach as it emphasizes the processes involved in the therapeutic relationship, which are crucial for treatment across all mental health diagnoses. Indeed, as noted by Wetterneck and Hart (2012), difficulties related to intimacy and interpersonal relationships crucially span a wide range of psychiatric disorders, and FAP adeptly addresses these aspects in its theoretical and practical framework. Moreover, Oshiro et al. (2021) argue that the foundational principles of FAP align with the tenets of Process-Based Therapy (PBT), presented by Hayes and Hoffman (2018) as an alternative to the limitations faced in the syndromic diagnostic model of the DSM (Diagnostic and Statistical Manual of Mental Disorders), further strengthening the current transdiagnostic movement. As Oshiro et al. (2021) analyze, FAP, by presenting a philosophical foundation consistent with a specific case formulation and proposing an understanding of what is functionally healthy and pathological regarding interpersonal relationships and intimacy, is stepping into the realm of PBTs.

The assessment and case formulation in FAP emphasize a functional description based on basic behavioral principles, through which the therapist will ideographically define (intrasubject assessment) the CRBs, taking into consideration the client's life history, reported issues, and also the behaviors that occur in session during the interaction with the therapist. As highlighted by Kanter et al. (2009), a DSM-based diagnosis is not a sufficient assessment strategy in FAP, as it lacks elements that guide specific interventions the therapist needs to target. Thus, an essential component in terms of assessment strategies in FAP is flexibility and adaptation, addressing the unique needs of each clinical case, which sets FAP apart from other standardized therapies.

According to Kanter et al. (2009), the assessment process in FAP is collaboratively built between therapist and client. This results in the recognition of behavioral patterns, which, when organized ideographically, will assist the therapist in: identifying when improvements occur in session; and making strategic and genuine choices in response to these improvements. The assessment in FAP does not aim to technically label the client's behavior, but rather, through the evaluative process, to identify relationships that aid in understanding why behaviors causing harm to the client are being maintained.

In other words, FAP does not propose an assessment and treatment protocol based on specific mental disorder diagnoses. According to Kanter et al. (2017), FAP is consistent with an ideographic analysis in which behaviors are described in functional rather than topographic terms, evaluated through the lens of the 5 Rules and classifications of CRBs. However, presenting it in these terms makes it challenging to standardize the treatment, as well as replicate procedures in clinical trial research. Consequently, research findings do not highlight FAP as an approach focused on psychiatric disorders due to the intrinsic characteristics of the approach.

The therapeutic goals in FAP, as noted by Oshiro et al. (2021), are not solely aimed at symptom reduction but also focus on clients building interpersonal repertoires of intimacy that serve as important protective factors in their daily lives. Consistent with these therapeutic expectations, the review conducted by Kanter et al. (2017) highlights that FAP techniques, when applied to individually defined behavioral problems, bring positive changes in these behaviors both within and outside the therapy session. These findings also provide evidence that the proposed mechanism of change in FAP (modeling improved behavior in session through contingent reinforcement by the therapist) is valid.

Even though it is not an approach focused on specific diagnoses, FAP has been chosen and successfully applied to a wide range of complaints (anxiety, depression, sexual problems, relationship difficulties, chronic pain, personality disorders, among others) according to López-Bermúdez et al. (2021), precisely due to its transdiagnostic nature focusing on processes inherent in the therapeutic relationship. According to these authors, who researched the efficacy of FAP in 10 clinical cases with different psychopathology diagnosis, the results demonstrated effectiveness in reducing the initial array of reported problems, as well as an improvement in their interpersonal repertoires perceived by the clients and also endorsed by their closest social network.

In that same vein, back in 2010, Kanter et al. (2010) proposed an integration of FAP with a broad spectrum of approaches (CBT, ACT, DBT, BA, among others), including a diverse client population (couples, teenagers, sexual minorities, groups, different cultures, among others). In this work, the authors explicitly illustrate how it's possible to expand the psychotherapy process based on the FAP framework. Particularly, by integrating FAP with CBT, Kohlenberg et al. (2010) point out that despite substantial evidence in standardized treatments like CBT, it's also known that standardization does not work for everyone and in every situation, making FAP a viable option in such cases.

In FAP—Enhanced Cognitive Therapy, as suggested by Kohlenberg et al. (2010), the gains from this integration bring an expansion of the rationale presented to clients about the cause of their problems. It also enhances standard CBT treatment by utilizing the therapeutic relationship as a live learning opportunity. The authors also emphasize the need for flexibility in providing a behavioral interpretation of cognitions. In relation to the CRBs, these can be either interpersonal (for example, when the client appears cold and distant in response to the therapist's care and attention) and/or cognitive CRBs (when the client believes they will be rejected by the therapist if they express dissatisfaction with something in therapy during a session). In both cases, there is an emphasis on the behavior that occurs in the here and now, through which the therapist will evaluate based on FAP principles to manage their interventions and propose homework assignments.

Intimacy as a Therapeutic Target and FAP's Contributions

As discussed in previous sections, intimacy holds clinical importance in FAP. When establishing it as a target in the therapeutic process, it's crucial to consider that clients often share deeply personal information. FAP therapists are encouraged to genuinely engage in these interactions with the aim of increasing intimacy between therapist and client. This, in turn, strengthens the therapeutic relationship, potentially impacting progress in treating interpersonal issues. Genuine interaction implies a relationship where the therapist may describe to the client the possible impacts that a revelation, such as the disclosure of a traumatic situation, has on the therapist. From the perspective of FAP, intense and powerful interactions, arising from naturally reinforcing exchanges, create a safe therapeutic environment for developing an enhanced interpersonal repertoire that can be generalized to the client's other relationships (Knott et al., 2015).

It's important to emphasize that even though self-disclosure is an element required within the repertoire of a FAP therapist, it should be done for the benefit of the client and functionally analyzed. This doesn't mean making indiscriminate disclosures or providing the client with the therapist's personal details to meet the therapist's needs (Tsai et al., 2009a). In other words, the therapist's self-disclosures, such as their reactions and feelings in response to the client's disclosures, are made with the therapeutic goal of encouraging/reinforcing the client's behavior to occur more frequently in the future.

FAP, due to its functional, idiographic, and essentially transdiagnostic nature, can be applied to a wide range of clinical complaints and different contexts (Kanter et al., 2010). However, as the literature exposes, its mechanism is inherently interpersonal, more frequently recommended as an approach aimed at clinical targets related to interpersonal functioning and issues arising from the intimacy process (Tsai et al., 2009b; Holman et al., 2017). Effectively, Wetterneck and Hart (2012) suggest FAP as an approach that could bridge a gap in transdiagnostic treatments within CBTs, particularly targeting interpersonal changes, especially focusing on intimacy as a therapeutic goal.

The identification of intimacy as a therapeutic target can be carried out when formulating the FAP case (Kanter et al., 2009), as well as when analyzing the client's complaints, reports and behavior in session from the perspective of the ACL Model (Holman et al., 2017; Maitland et al., 2017) and/or from the interpersonal classes proposed by the FIAT model (Callaghan, 2006). Below we bring a formulation of a real case attended by the first author together with some interventions and analyses on the therapeutic process guided by the FAP perspective. The client consented to the publication of his data, and information that could expose or identify him was changed and/or suppressed.

Example of a Clinical Case

When constructing a FAP Case Formulation, Kanter et al. (2009) list several essential topics that the therapist should investigate and seek to answer in order to formulate hypotheses, as well as define CRBs and their therapeutic intervention plan. Below, we explore these topics (highlighted in underline), incorporating information about the client named here as Fábio (fictitious name).

Relevant life history: Fábio is 34 years old, single, and did not complete high school. He has been working at the same place for 15 years and lives with his parents. He describes a humble childhood with limited financial resources, growing up in a rural area with few social interactions. He felt ashamed to go to school in old clothes and did not finish high school due to shame and the fear of exposure in situations that were required (e.g., presenting a project, asking questions in class). He describes himself as a very shy child and continues to struggle with shame and difficulties in social interactions. His parents have low education and poor interpersonal skills, which did not foster the development of a satisfactory interpersonal repertoire in Fábio. The client reports difficulties in starting conversations, making friends, attending social events, and has never had a romantic relationship, although he currently desires to establish social, friendship, and romantic relationships.

O1s (Outside or daily life problematic behaviors): Difficulty expressing opinions to colleagues and subordinates in the workplace. Avoids potential conflict situations. Struggles to make requests or express needs, leading to overload both at work and in personal life. Avoids leaving home due to fear of saying or doing something wrong, for example, in a restaurant. Feels ashamed to approach women, hindering his desire for a romantic relationship. Struggles to initiate simple conversations in stores or during phone calls, for instance. Experiences high levels of anxiety in all these problematic situations, leading to avoidance and subsequent sadness due to not achieving his goals (assertiveness at work, social and romantic relationships).

Problematic beliefs: "If I make a mistake, they'll think I'm stupid. My shame prevents me from doing what I want. Nobody will like me because of my appearance."

Maintaining variables of the problems: The work schedule makes it difficult for him to accept invitations on weekends and have contact with more people. He lives with overprotective parents. He avoids emotional discomfort by not exposing himself, which limits his repertoire and causes him to avoid social situations and, consequently, intimacy in relationships.

Advantages and positive points: Has financial independence. Strong motivation for treatment. Has made progress in work-related complaints. Is motivated and engaged in treatment. Accepts agreed-upon tasks and makes an effort to accomplish them.

CRB1s: Difficulty expressing concerns during sessions (speaking rapidly or sometimes getting stuck when trying to speak or providing very brief statements without elaboration); Rigid body posture with a frightened look, rapid breathing, blushing on the face, and other noticeable parts of the body (neck) along with statements like "I'm very ashamed in front of you"; Leaving more challenging subjects to discuss towards the end of the session and thereby speaking less about them; Passivity during sessions: not taking the initiative to introduce a topic, often leaving this role to the therapist; Accepting changes in session time requested by the therapist without considering their impact on his routine.

CRB2s: Recognition of his emotions during the session ("This is how I feel when I have to talk to someone"); Staying in the emotional experience while interacting with the therapist; Providing a more detailed description of his emotions, thoughts, and body sensations; Self-disclosure of situations in which (in his perception) he might be judged; Suggesting relevant topics during the session; Requesting a change in the schedule considering his needs, even if he is afraid of displeasing or causing inconvenience to the therapist.

O2s (Outside or daily life target/improved behaviors): Recognizing his emotions and needs. Expressing his needs and requests in his relationships with coworkers. Accepting invitations to go out. Allowing himself to tolerate uncomfortable situations (like talking to a stranger or the cashier at the market) for the purpose of advancing his objectives. Experiencing new situations, such as traveling.

Therapy goals: Build and strengthen interpersonal skills that benefit him in both work-related and personal relationships.

T1s (Therapist in-session problematic behaviors): Overly leading the session, facilitating client avoidance by not taking the initiative and developing the conversation; Staying excessively within the content of the client's issues, avoiding entering the interpersonal process to prevent evoking emotional discomfort in the client; Seeking quick solutions to the problems presented, avoiding experiencing the emotions arising from the situation.

T2s (Therapist in-session target/improved behaviors): Tolerate silences to evoke behaviors of initiative in starting and developing the subject with F.; Evoke and stay within F.'s emotional experience; Express security and validation in the face of the client's difficulties when exposing themselves in the session.

The therapist noted (Rule 1) that Fábio presented a significantly deficient repertoire regarding the identification of his feelings, needs, and values, coupled with a high level of anxiety in social interaction situations, leading him to avoid such scenarios. Therefore, the initial strategy concerning his CRBs was to evoke (Rule 2) and reinforce (Rule 3) as many responses as possible where he expressed his opinions, feelings, and needs. Regarding this process, it was necessary to invest in successive modeling (Rule 3), checking the effect of these on the client's behavior (Rule 4) due to the wide range of responses that needed to be modeled into his repertoire.

Gradually, these interventions strengthened and increased the frequency of his CRB2 in interaction with the therapist, which has also allowed for establishing parallels (Rule 5) between problematic situations in his life and the therapy process. Homework assignments (Rule 5) needed to be planned according to the level of difficulty the client reported tolerating and the risks he was encouraged to take in his daily relationships. In this sense, even though he couldn't control how his contexts would receive his behavioral changes, it was important to carefully assess so that a repertoire learned and encouraged in session, when attempting to be generalized, wouldn't be punished. Therefore, we planned small tasks in which the client gradually challenged himself. Among these, greeting people in his daily activities, making necessary work-related calls (which he avoided), and accepting invitations to dinner at a colleague's house whom he knew. Initially, these were situations he avoided, and with the support of the therapeutic process, he managed to expose himself, despite feeling emotional discomfort. Alongside the in-session interventions of evocation and consequentiality to strengthen his interpersonal repertoire, more complex tasks were stipulated for the client, such as expressing his opinion in a probable conflict situation.

Regarding daily life goals and therapy objectives, the client has achieved significant success, although there are still some unmet goals (such as having a romantic relationship, for example). Initially, work relationships were identified as therapeutic targets, which the client reports to be progressing. For instance, the client feels more confident and successful in expressing opinions, setting boundaries, addressing work-related issues, making phone calls, delegating tasks, among others. Another therapeutic gain was that for the first time in 15 years, during vacation, he traveled and explored a new city. Additionally, the client resumed studying to complete high school and plans to pursue further courses. He attributes this newfound openness to therapy, something previously unimaginable and strongly avoided. The client continues in therapy as therapeutic goals are being refined based on his progress and tolerance for emotionally challenging situations.

Conclusion

FAP is a third-generation/wave therapy within Cognitive and Behavioral Therapies, which is based on the assumption that the therapeutic relationship shares functional similarities with other relationships in the client's daily life, and through this, more effective and healthier repertoires can be modeled for clients' lives. For emphasizing the processes involved in the therapeutic relationship, which are important for treatment across all mental health diagnoses, FAP is also a transdiagnostic approach (Holman et al., 2017).

In contrast to standardized protocols that follow a specific order of intervention, in transdiagnostic treatment, the intervention is directed and adapted based on the dysfunctional coping strategies most commonly used by the client in reality. Thus, for a transdiagnostic approach, there is an increasing focus on interventions that seek a broader view of the client and encompass the existing psychological processes from a non-pathologizing and ideographic perspective that promotes progress.

FAP masterfully introduces an assessment and intervention proposal focused on interactions established through the therapeutic relationship, particularly in issues involving the process of intimacy and its resulting problems. This enhances therapeutic gains beyond closed intervention protocols. The chapter also presented a case where the results made it clear how valid this clinical reasoning is, validating the contributions of FAP to the development of more transdiagnostic interventions within CBTs.

References

Callaghan, G. M. (2006). The Functional Idiographic Assessment Template (FIAT) system: For use with interpersonally-based interventions including Functional Analytic Psychotherapy (FAP) and FAP-enhanced treatments. *The Behavior Analyst Today, 7*(3), 357–398. https://doi.org/10.1037/h0100160

Cordova, J. V., & Scott, R. L. (2001). Intimacy: A behavioral interpretation. *The Behavior Analyst, 24*, 75–86.

Hartmann, A. V.-B., Oshiro, C. K. B., & Vartanian, J. F. (2018). Psicoterapia analítica funcional (FAP): mudança clínica evocada e modelada pela vivência terapêutica. In *Psicologia clínica da graduação à pós-graduação*. Atheneu.

Hayes, S. C., & Hoffman, S. G. (2018). *Process based CBT: Core clinical competencies in evidence-based treatment*. Context Press/New Harbinger Publications.

Holman, G., Kanter, J., Tsai, M., & Kohlenberg, R. (2017). *Functional analytic psychotherapy made simple: A practical guide to therapeutic relationships*. New Harbinger Publications.

Holt-Lunstad, J., Smith, T. B., & Layton, J. B. (2010). Social relationships and mortality risk: A meta-analytic review. *PLoS Medicine, 7*(7), e1000316. https://doi.org/10.1371/journal.pmed.1000316

Kanter, J., Weeks, C., Bonow, J., Landes, J., Callaghan, G., & Follete, C. (2009). Assessment and case conceptualization. In M. Tsai, R. J. Kohlenberg, J. W. Kanter, B. Kohlenberg, W. C. Follette, & G. M. Callaghan (Eds.), *A guide to functional analytic psychotherapy: Awareness, courage, love and behaviorism* (pp. 37–59). Springer Science & Business Media.

Kanter, J., Tsai, M., & Kohlenberg, R. (Eds.). (2010). *The practice of functional analytic psychotherapy*. Springer Science Business Media, LLC.

Kanter, J., Manbeck, K., Kuczynski, A., Maitland, D., Villas-Bôas, A., & Reyes, M. (2017). A comprehensive review of research on functional analytic psychotherapy. *Clinical Psychology Review, 58*. https://doi.org/10.1016/j.cpr.2017.09.010

Knott, L. E., Wetterneck, C. T., Derr, D., & Tolentino, R. (2015). A functional analytic perspective of therapist intimacy in and out of session. *International Journal of Behavioral Consultation and Therapy, 9*(4), 6–10.

Kohlenberg, R. J., & Tsai, M. (1991). *Functional analytic psychotherapy: Creating intense and curative therapeutic relationships*. Plenum.

Kohlenberg, R., Kanter, J., Tsai, M., & Weeks, C. (2010). FAP and cognitive behavior therapy. In J. W. Kanter, M. Tsai, & R. J. Kohlenberg (Eds.), *The practice of functional analytic psychotherapy* (pp. 11–30). Springer Science Business Media, LLC.

Leahy. (2002). A model of emotional schemas. *Cognitive and Behavioral Practice, 9*(3), 177–190.

López-Bermúdez, M. A., Ferro-García, R., Calvillo-Mazarro, M., & Valero-Aguayo, L. (2021). Importance of the therapeutic relationship: Efficacy of functional analytic psychotherapy with different problems. *Clínica y Salud, 32*(3), 103–109. https://doi.org/10.5093/clysa2020a32

Maitland, D., Kanter, J., Manbeck, K., & Kuczynski, A. (2017). Relationship science informed clinically relevant behaviors in functional analytic psychotherapy: The awareness, courage, and love model. *Journal of Contextual Behavioral Science, 6*(4), 347–359., ISSN 2212-1447. https://doi.org/10.1016/j.jcbs.2017.07.002

McKay, Fanning, & Zurita. (2011). *Mind and emotions: A universal treatment for emotional disorders*. New Harbinger Publications.

Oshiro, Vartanian, Sartor, & Silva. (2021). A Psicoterapia Analítica Funcional (FAP). In C. K. B. Oshiro, & T. A. S. Ferreira (orgs), *Terapias Contextuais Comportamentais: análise funcional e prática clínica*. Manole.

Reis, H. T. (2007). Steps toward the ripening of relationship science. *Personal Relationships, 14*(1), 1–23. https://doi.org/10.1111/j.1475-6811.2006.00139.x

Reis, H. T., & Patrick, B. C. (1996). Attachment and intimacy: Component processes. In E. T. Higgins & A. W. Kruglanski (Eds.), *Social psychology: Handbook of basic principles* (pp. 523–563). Guilford Press.

Reis, H. T., & Shaver, P. (1988). Intimacy as an interpersonal process. In S. W. Duck (Ed.), *Handbook of personal relationships* (pp. 367–389). Wiley.

Sauer-Zavala, S., Gutner, C. A., Farchione, T. J., Boettcher, H. T., Bullis, J. R., & Barlow, D. H. (2017). Current definitions of "transdiagnostic" in treatment development: A search for consensus. *Behavior Therapy, 48*, 128–138.

Tsai, M., Kohlenberg, B., Kanter, W., & Waltz, J. (2009a). Therapeutic technique: The five rules. In M. Tsai, R. J. Kohlenberg, J. Kanter, B. Kohlenberg, W. Follette, & G. Callaghan (Eds.), *A guide to functional analytic psychotherapy: Awareness, courage, love and behaviorism* (pp. 61–102). New York: Springer.

Tsai, M., Kohlenberg, R. J., Kanter, J. W., Kohlenberg, B., Follette, W. C., & Callaghan, G. M. (2009b). *A guide to functional analytic psychotherapy: Awareness, courage, love and behaviorism*. New York: Springer Science & Business Media.

Tsai, M., Yoo, D., Hardebeck, E. J., Loudon, M. P., & Kohlenberg, R. J. (2019, January 24). Creating safe, evocative, attuned, and mutually vulnerable therapeutic beginnings: Strategies from functional analytic psychotherapy. *Psychotherapy*. Advance online publication. https://doi.org/10.1037/pst0000203

Wetterneck, C. T., & Hart, J. (2012). Intimacy is a transdiagnostic problem for cognitive behavior therapy: Functional analytical psychotherapy is a solution. *International Journal of Behavioral and Consultation Therapy, 7*, 2–3.

Chapter 5
Mindfulness-Based Cognitive Therapy as a Tool to Manage Emotional and Psychological Distress

Vitor Friary

Introduction

Mindfulness has been widely defined as the individual's capacity to show up in the present moment non-judgmentally and able to accept experiences as they are. It has been a central practice in a different number of fields, such as yoga and meditation traditions throughout the world, and in the past decades have been used in more secular settings as a health and clinical psychology intervention. There's compelling evidence that mindfulness practices and skills help to reduce psychopathology in a wide range of clinical populations, helping to lessen the impact of psychological suffering, across a varied number of psychological disorders (Bach & Hayes, 2002; Linehan et al., 1999; Lynch et al., 2003).

Mindfulness skills are central components of the Mindfulness-based Cognitive Therapy (MBCT) protocol and this chapter shows how these are can be used to treat anxiety and depression related symptoms from a transdiagnostic perspective. To show this, firstly I will present what key processes are at play that contribute to the maintenance and aggravation of psychological suffering, then I will share with readers real case examples of how to use these skills in order to undermine these.

Brief History of the Development of MBCT

Mindfulness-Based Cognitive Therapy (MBCT) is a therapeutic approach that combines principles of cognitive therapy with mindfulness practices and was developed in the 1990s by clinical psychologists Zindel Segal, Mark Williams, and John Teasdale. Initially, the developers of MBCT were interested in finding ways to

V. Friary (✉)
Centre for Mindfulness in Brazil, Rio de Janeiro, Brazil

A. C. Ornelas (ed.), *Transdiagnostic Approaches in Cognitive Behavioral Therapy*, https://doi.org/10.1007/978-3-031-63494-9_5

prevent the recurrence of depressive episodes in individuals who had experienced multiple episodes of major depression.

MBCT integrated mindfulness practices, inspired by Jon Kabat-Zinn's Mindfulness-Based Stress Reduction (MBSR) 8-week program, with principles and activities of cognitive behavior therapy. Initially the MBSR program had a wider focus on being a generalized form of health intervention mostly focused on patients with chronic health conditions dealing with stress. On the other hand, MBCT founders hypothesized that by combining these two approaches, individuals could develop skills to break the cycle of depressive relapse, given that research at that stage already found that the more episodes of depression a person would have along their lives, the higher the chances of relapsing.

Research studies conducted by the founders and others supported the efficacy of MBCT in preventing the recurrence of depressive episodes. This evidence contributed to the growing popularity of MBCT within the mental health community. Over the years, MBCT has been adapted and applied beyond depression, addressing a range of mental health challenges.

The MBCT's structured 8-week program has become a hallmark of its approach, emphasizing the cultivation of mindfulness skills to interrupt automatic cognitive reactivity and teaching individuals to observe reactivity when it shows up, as well as holding and letting go softly of negative and dysfunctional thoughts. By encouraging a non-judgmental awareness to changes in mood and of the present moment from a wider view, MBCT empowers individuals to respond more skillfully to stressors, reducing the risk of relapse.

Today, MBCT stands as a prominent example of the integration of mindfulness practices into evidence-based psychological therapies. Its evolution reflects a commitment to addressing the complexities of mental health, offering individuals a proactive means of managing and preventing recurrent depressive episodes. Key transdiagnostic psychopathological processes addressed by MBCT interventions.

Mindlessness

This is by far one of the key processes that may prevent patients from getting unstuck from their relapsing cycles of emotional distress, and one that can easily be overlooked during real clinical sessions. Living in auto-pilot mode, or mindlessly navigating through daily life without conscious awareness, can have profound negative impacts on psychological wellbeing and on the maintenance of distress. This process is characterized by a lack of attention to present moment experience, a failure to engage with one's surroundings, specially making little use of sensory perception (Friary, 2018).

One of the primary negative impacts is the erosion of genuine connections with oneself and others. Mindless living often leads to a disconnection from one's emotions and an inability to understand the underlying causes of psychological distress. Individuals may find themselves trapped in a cycle of routine and habit and foster feelings of emptiness, loneliness, and a sense of purposelessness, contributing to increased psychological suffering.

Moreover, mindless living may exacerbate stress and anxiety. When individuals operate on auto-pilot, they are more likely to succumb to the pressures of daily life without adequately processing or managing stressors. This can lead to chronic stress, emotional exhaustion, and, ultimately, the development or exacerbation of mental health disorders.

In the absence of mindful awareness, individuals may also struggle with decision-making and problem-solving. Mindless living hampers cognitive flexibility and creative thinking, making it challenging to adapt to new situations or find innovative solutions to life's challenges. This cognitive rigidity can heighten feelings of frustration, helplessness, and a diminished sense of control over one's life circumstances.

Furthermore, mindless living may contribute to a diminished sense of self-esteem and self-worth. When individuals fail to engage with their passions, values, and personal growth, they may experience a lack of fulfillment and a sense of stagnation. This, in turn, can lead to feelings of inadequacy, self-doubt, and a pervasive sense of dissatisfaction.

Monitoring of Discrepancies

Both Mark Williams and Zindel Segal's contribution prior to the development of MBCT was really important. Williams and Segal's work, based on the self-discrepancy theory (Higgins, 1987), focused on how individuals who have experienced depression tend to have a heightened sensitivity to discrepancies between their current experiences and their expectations or standards, hence always comparing an 'idealized' state of wellbeing, usually of past lived experiences, with how things are 'in the moment' and how it should be different. This monitoring of discrepancies process often involves a focused attention to unwanted private experiences (thoughts, feelings, and bodily sensations) accompanied by judgement related cognitions of how things should be like instead. Evaluations of private experiences (awfulizing and complaining) often prevents the patient to see clearly the ever-changing nature of human experiences, and that thoughts, feelings and sensations are never *everlasting* as often seen during the moments of crisis. Reacting to unwanted stressful inner and outer experiences with judging and evaluating cognitions paradoxically reactivate unwanted related mood, which can lead to an aggravation of psychological distress overall.

Although the monitoring of discrepancies above has been understudied in the context of the transdiagnostic process, my experience in conducting over 140 MBCT intervention groups, with a huge variety of different cases and diagnosis, leads me to argue that the monitoring of discrepancies is present no matter what the condition may be. At the core of any psychological distress resides the urge to see this process end, to have it stopped and reverted back to how 'things used to be' before the crisis reported in psychotherapy. Might it be panic disorder, obsessive compulsive disorder diagnosis, or an experience of trauma, the mind innately activates cognitions of comparison and discrepancies with another 'more pleasant' experience of life. One could argue that one's mind does not even need to have a particular diagnosis for monitoring discrepancies, because that is just what mind's do.

Cognitive Reactivity and Cognitive Fusion

Another important contribution for the development of the MBCT protocol was Teasdale's take on cognitive vulnerability in what he called the differential activation hypothesis. This refers to the ease with which maladaptive cognitive processes and content triggered by mild mood change in psychological distress, known as *cognitive reactivity*, can help predict depression recurrence in remitted depressives. In other words, the degree to which an individual's mood change can influence the activation of negative thinking patterns, and in turn how these recurrent negative thinking patterns can further aggravate psychological distress. For the developers of MBCT, when individuals who have a history of depression encounter stress or negative events, they may be more prone to reactivate thought patterns with more negative content when compared to the larger non-clinical population (Cladder-Micus et al., 2018).

The tendency to think that unwanted private experiences '*may never change*' or '*never go away*' or are '*unsolvable and unbearable*' are often main themes that permeate the cognitive reactivity process. The patient looks at his psychological experience literally *through* these thoughts, and therefore jumps to the conclusion that the way psychological distress work is the way he or she thinks they do as oppose to how they *actually are*.

Getting caught by thoughts and *fusing* with them is a cognitive process known as *cognitive fusion* and is largely associated with the individual's difficulties in letting emotional experience just come and go, more lightly. This process deepens the effect of cognitive reactivity and have a more negative impact on the patient's capacity to feel emotions and mood changes as they really are.

Let's deepen our understanding of the cognitive fusion process. It involves the way individuals perceive their thoughts, particularly when thoughts are considered absolute truths. In such instances, emotions and behaviors become intricately tied to the certainty attributed to these cognitions (Hayes et al., 2011). In simpler terms, cognitive fusion involves experiencing thoughts as undeniable truths, where individuals are dominated by, wholeheartedly believe in, and strictly adhere to their thoughts. This inclination towards cognitive fusion often comes at the expense of mental decentering, wherein thoughts are viewed as mental contents without necessitating externalized behaviors or expressed actions (Hayes et al., 2011, 2012).

Consistent findings from previous research have indicated a positive association between cognitive fusion and various symptoms, including shame, social anxiety, depression, obsessive-compulsive disorder, devaluation of physical image in eating disorders, and psychological distress (Faustino et al., 2023). Furthermore, cognitive fusion has been shown to exhibit positive correlations with more structural mental variables, such as early maladaptive schemas and dysfunctional interpersonal cycles (Faustino & Vasco, 2020a).

Conversely, cognitive fusion displays negative correlations with psychological well-being, the regulation of psychological needs (Faustino & Vasco, 2020a, b), as well as metacognition (Faustino et al., 2019). Additionally, emotional regulation difficulties have been found to be negatively correlated with cognitive fusion across two independent samples, regardless of diagnosis (Faustino, 2021). Consequently, prior research underscores the presence of cognitive fusion in both non-clinical and sub-clinical samples, providing further support for this assertion (Cookson et al., 2019).

As it could be argued that cognitive fusion is a transdiagnostic process (Faustino et al., 2023) one may also observe cognitive reactivity from the same perspective. The latter does not predict depression recurrence in remitted depressives alone, but predicts in general the remission of any disorder. As every time an individual experiences a recurrent crisis or a worsening in symptoms, this is often associated with very negative cognitions, for example, of things 'never changing' or 'suffering never going away'. This way of reacting, one may argue, is cognitive reactivity, that in turn, lead to the aggravation of negative affect and keeps the individual stuck in a loop hole of psychological distress no matter the diagnosis.

Experiential Avoidance

In addition to the contributions of the above cognitive processes in the maintenance of psychological distress there is also extensive empirical evidence that points to the prevalence of Experiential Avoidance (EA) as a functional dimension in various psychological issues. EA is characterized as the "phenomenon that occurs when a person is unwilling to remain in contact with particular private psychological experiences (e.g., bodily sensations, emotions, thoughts, memories, behavioral predispositions) and takes steps to alter the form or frequency of these events and the contexts that occasion them" through the means of a wide variety of avoidance strategies (Hayes et al., 1996, p. 1154).

Although avoiding unwanted inner experiences may provide short-term relief, it paradoxically heightens distress over a long-term period (Bardeen, 2015). When this avoidance strategy solidifies into an inflexible behavioral pattern, it detrimentally impacts the individual's functionality across various life domains. By running away and resisting to unwanted experiences, individuals' distance themselves from pertinent life conditions, simultaneously losing contact with the very circumstances that could, and should, foster change. Consequently, distress intensifies, getting the person stuck in a loop of avoidance.

Experiential avoidance is hypothesized to play a pivotal role in the origin, persistence, and modification of various forms of psychopathology, emerging as a core vulnerability factor for emotional distress. Laboratory studies illustrate that experiential avoidance amplifies anxiety symptomatology even in individuals without a history of anxiety-related disorders (Ruiz, 2010). Regarding depression, theoretical accounts posit that EA modifies an individual's emotional experience, consequently escalating psychological distress and worsening depressive symptoms. Studies involving adults consistently indicate a robust positive correlation between EA and depression, especially among women with affective disorders (Spinhoven et al., 2014).

Rumination and Worrying

Rumination is a form of repetitive negative thinking (RNT) over the potential causes, meanings, and consequences of negative life events after an individual has encountered them (Nolen-Hoeksema et al., 2008) while worry is another RNT, rather focused on possible or imagined *future* uncertainties, risks, and catastrophes and how an individual would cope with these if they were to occur. Rumination and worry are transdiagnostic processes, each associated with symptoms of both anxiety and depression and often co-occurring in the same individual. Both rumination and worry have repeatedly been implicated in the onset, severity, maintenance, and increased relapse risk of both depression and anxiety disorders (Watkins & Roberts, 2020). Rumination and worry are highly correlated and share more similarities than differences, with thought content and temporal orientation the only consistently replicated variation.

Considered a maladaptive strategy for regulating emotions in response to negative life situations, rumination and worrying hinder effective coping with negative emotions (Crane, 2023). When faced with stressful events, individuals often employ various emotion regulation strategies to enhance their emotional well-being. Successful emotion regulation can contribute to improved mental health and better interpersonal relationships. However, a meta-analysis revealed that rumination, for example, is a more harmful emotion regulation approach compared to other strategies like acceptance, problem resolution, reappraisal, or suppression (Aldao et al., 2010). Rumination and worrying are also known as the process in which the patient gets "stuck" on certain thoughts or mental patterns, and may find it challenging to disengage from these repetitive cognitive processes.

RNT's may perpetuate the patient's mood changes activation, extending the period the crisis may last. It could also be argued that both are a form of aversion or experiential avoidance, as it may also prevent individuals from getting in contact with the embodied sensations of the inevitable suffering of how things were and the uncertainty of how things could turn out to be. As the patient keeps thinking about the unwanted troubling situations, he is not actually *experiencing* these difficulties as they actually are, that is, painful sensations that rise and fall naturally as time passes, and that don't actually need to be *solved* but rather experienced as the natural process of life: memories or uncertainties. In Fig. 5.1 it is possible to see how these processes might work at feeding back the patient's psychological distress and symptomatology.

Essential Mindfulness Skills in MBCT

The way that individuals process their private internal experiences is directly related to the extent that they will be vulnerable to an aggravation of their emotional and psychological distress (Crane, 2023). The purpose of the skills that MBCT interventions present to individuals is to help them work effectively with thoughts, emotions and sensations that arise in times of distress, so that they can stop getting stuck by them. Essentially the mindfulness processes described below and the perpetuation or maintenance of depression or anxiety symptoms are incompatible.

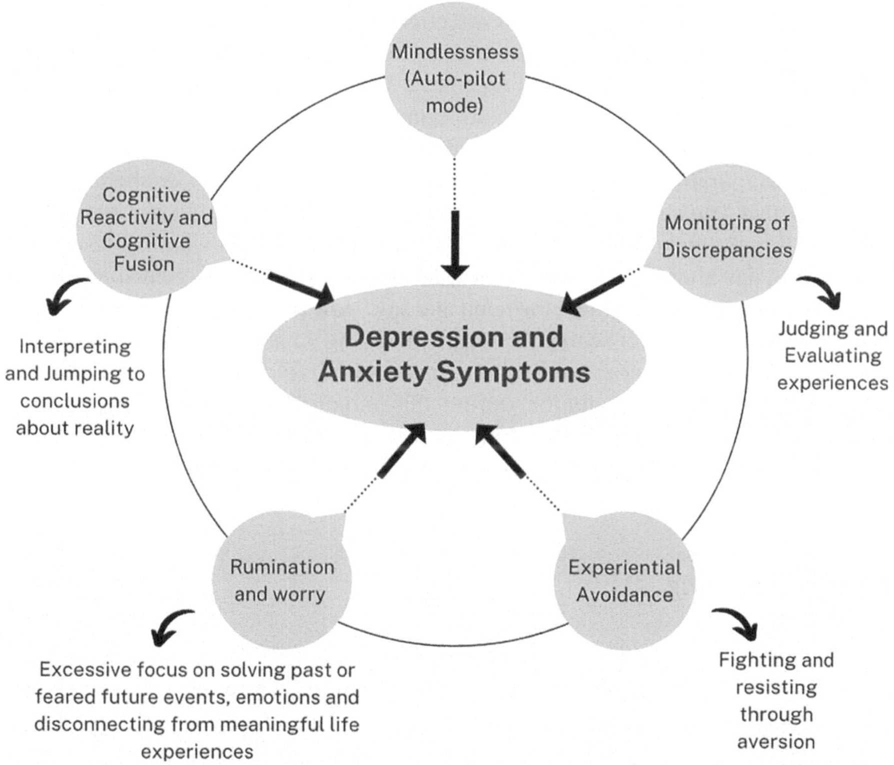

Fig. 5.1 Psychological distress and symptomatology

Attentional Training

Attentional training is an essential skill embedded in the majority of the MBCT therapy curriculum and taught throughout the program during the guided mindfulness interventions. Patients are taught that attention naturally drifts away from present sensorial experiences, and that we are often stuck in cognitive processes such as worrying, remembering, ruminating, brooding, planning, fantasizing. During the mindfulness interventions clinicians teach patients to notice where attention is and where it goes, and to deliberately bring attention back to a chosen focus point (seeing, touching, smelling, hearing, flavoring and the decentered observation of mental experiences). This is a crucial tool because it teaches people that there is choice in the way of relating to internal experience, and that is possible to purposefully move attention from one point to another. Moreover, this attention training prepares patients to know when to bring attention to and away from experience, when to be present, and when to let go, to notice the next experience arising in the present moment.

This skill is particularly present during exercises like the *raisin meditation* that is a first step in teaching patients what mindfulness is: *a present moment awareness with a non-judgmental attitude of openness and curiosity.* In our clinic, patients are taught that it is possible to invite out attention to the present moment, and choose purposefully to be present on a day-to-day life, holding lightly some unique attitudes like curiosity, receptivity and openness, and that this can be practiced with a day-to-day routine, like eating. More importantly, this exercise is teaching patients patiently to bring this same type of awareness to troubling thoughts and feelings, but first we need to train attention and make attention somewhat more deliberate.

During this "*raisin*" intervention it is common for therapists to ask patients to take attention throughout their five senses, mindfully observing what is present and deliberating pay attention to what is showing up in each sense. Therapist might ask clients to place the one raisin on the hand and say "now placing your attention deliberately on the felt sense of seeing this raisin. Noticing what is present. *As you notice your attention moving away from seeing, just noticing and bringing your attention gently back*". This last invitation during this mindfulness exercise is preparing patients to take more control over their attention, so they can later use this skill in more useful ways of dealing, for example, with worrying and ruminating.

Mindful Noticing

In general patients will come to the clinic with a set of beliefs about emotional and mental experiences. Usually, thoughts, emotions and sensations are viewed as either good or bad states of experiences. *Mindful noticing* is about noticing private internal experiences as they are as opposed to judging or evaluating them. It does not mean noticing something unpleasant and pretending it isn't, but rather noticing what is and leaving judgment and evaluations as simply thoughts that can be gently observed and released.

During the guided skills building exercises, such as the *awareness of breathing* practice for example, where we get patients to notice their breathing flowing and out of the body, the patient is asked to notice thoughts, feelings and sensations along the practice just as passing experiences. Bringing mindfulness awareness to these flowing experiences means creating space for what is present, and observing internal private experiences changing moment by moment. This can be particularly helpful in moments of emotional distress. Being able to notice psychological experiences from a distance means to *decenter* away from what is present, and simply becoming a *good observer*, and nothing more than a gentle and open observer. Consequently, patients learn that mindfully noticing experiences, these thoughts, feelings and sensations can change. Learning the skill to hold each moment in awareness as it is with a non-judgmental attitude make it less possible individuals get entangled by the vicious circle of psychological distress.

As patients let go of evaluating experiences as good or bad, right or wrong, better or worse, and simply notice moments for what they are, that is that moments are simply moments, a sense of confidence and trust grows in how to manage mood, otherwise experienced as overwhelming.

Decentering and Defusion

Non-depressed individuals or those without an anxiety disorder diagnosis also feel unwanted stressful sensations and emotions from time to time, and even may have dysfunctional thoughts popping into the mind. At our clinic we invite patients to learn, through thoughts and feelings daily records, that mood and thinking can vary immensely in a single day. The reality is that mood and thinking change all the time. But in this case, people are just able to decenter from these thoughts and feelings more rapidly and instantly, that is, able to get unstuck. On the other hand, depressed or anxious patients tend to get stuck in dysfunctional thoughts and mood change more easily. This can have them trapped in a vicious cycle of distress and reactivity, perpetuating psychological suffering that the skill of *decentering* can help to break.

Decentering or defusing from thoughts, feelings and sensations literally means to get unstuck from its center, and to see these as merely events of the human experience. Situations bring about reactions, that is just what situations do. When patients learn to decenter or defuse from reactions, they recognize they are merely the observer of these, and start to notice these from a less personal perspective. This can help soothe the process and aid patients towards holding experiences more lightly, and view them as an ongoing flow of human experiences.

Additionally, decentering and defusing mean to notice thoughts in particular in a less literate way. Learning to observe thoughts like "*no matter what I do, nothing changes*" for example, as merely a block of words and sounds, and events that pop into mind that can actually simply be held, non-judgmentally in mind for the time that it lasts, without actually trying to solve its issue or try to modify it with 'better' or 'more positive' thoughts. Learning to observe thoughts in a less literate way can help patients see negative painful thoughts from a more manageable place.

Recognizing Mental Habits

During the MBCT interventions patients are guided by the therapist to see clearly how thoughts popping in the mind can trigger a number of emotional, and physical reactions. The tendency of the mind to judge, criticize, ruminate, worry, find someone to blame, shaming, catastrophize, among other idiosyncratic habits of thinking that may directly linked to the mental condition they present on treatment, when recognized can more effectively be dealt with. These mental habits can further feed uncomfortable life events with more discomfort, as thinking patterns keep reactivating distressful emotional states. Once we teach these skills of recognizing mental habits, and this happens for example during the guided practices, patients learn to stop this vicious cycle. This interruption can lead patients to see the stressful situations from a different angle and most importantly can help soothe their painful mood (Akbari et al., 2022).

Additionally, getting to know what are the typical thoughts that show up in the individual's mind during recurrent life stressful events can help them notice reactivity piling up just in time to prevent falling into cycles of unhelpful ways to manage these situations and therefore preventing symptoms to worsen.

Gently Relating to Bodily Sensations

When patients are experiencing mood changes and psychological distress, they rarely stop to come into actually feel their bodies. There is too much attention given to cognition in psychological distress and little attention to actually sensing distress as it actually happens in the body. This can usually raise up the frequency and intensity of negative disturbing thoughts, which can in turn feed the unpleasant experience with more unpleasant experience, making the situation feel *unbearable*. During mindfulness exercises, especially in MBCT, patients are invited to recognize when painful and uncomfortable private internal experiences show up. This can happen in two different ways, either instructions for patients to observe when mood changes along the guided practice (boredom, agitation, sadness, worrying, planning the future, ruminating the past, etc.), or therapist may actually ask patients to bring a troubling event to mind that may have caused a certain amount of emotional distress in the past week or so.

Additionally, therapists guide patients to noticing where emotional pain actually is in the *body*, locating it, and further instructions into staying present with these sensations with an attitude of non-judging. Breathing gently with the sensations just as they are, as the air comes and out of this place, and to notice moment by moment what happens. At the same time releasing away expectations of *should's* and *shouldn'ts*, and just staying present gently and being a good observer. Further instructions of letting thoughts just be in the background, and be released out with the outbreath, can further attune patients into this skill of attending to intense emotional bodily sensations, and decentering from thoughts, that otherwise have the tendency to aggravate distress. As we move toward sensations of emotional distress in the body, and release from thoughts that feed more pain into the situations we are living, we might become aware of how experiences do change, and as the sensations change, we may be more prone to find more helpful ways of dealing with life's challenges that are being presented. Moreover, individuals who practice gently relating to bodily sensations of discomfort and emotional pain may actually learn that depression and anxiety symptoms are neither permanent nor fixed states.

Applying Mindfulness Interventions

There are some key interventions in the 8-week MBCT therapy program, and I will present here some of them, with a clear understanding of what are the main learning therapeutic goals for each one of them, and real case examples of how they have been applied in our clinic. Although the MBCT program is essentially a group intervention, the interventions can be used as part of individual psychotherapy.

Doing Something with Mindful Awareness

This is commonly known in the MBCT program as the *raisin meditation*, but in our clinic, we name it different, as it is interesting that patients fix in the mind the learning that this exercise is directed towards all type of situations and activities of our daily lives. Mindfulness can be applied to all types of situations and daily activities. It is an exercise where we intend to teach patients the difference between living mindlessly and living mindfully, and what are the main characteristics of this type of awareness. Moreover, individuals learn how frequent they actually function on auto-pilot mode, and how mindful awareness can actually reveal never before aspect of an experience, and how mindful awareness can actually *change* experience. This is particularly helpful because we want to present to patients how mindfulness can also be helpful a way to meet internal private experiences, including discomfort. Finally, this exercise can help us teach patients to notice how rapidly the mind can react with thoughts, feelings and sensations in the handling of simple tasks like *eating a raisin*.

See below a basic script for running this experiment in session with a client, followed by an exploratory dialogue, which in the MBCT program it is known as *inquiry*. You will need a small piece of nut, or you will need one raisin for running this, and you will be placing this in your patient's palm of the hand:

Therapist: "Now place this small *object* in the palm of your hand, and let's explore it, patiently, moment by moment, with all our senses. Firstly, exploring it with sight. Seeing this object and noticing it as if it was the very first time you will seeing this. What do you see? What colors does it have? What about its shape? Is there something present that you have never seen before? Exploring what you see, with a curious mind, leaving thoughts and judgments that may rise in the mind, simply fall away with your out-breath, and just remaining present with the felt sense of seeing. Now shifting your attention to your sense of touch. Touching this object slowly, and sensing it texture. What are your fingers feelings as you run them softly over the surface of this object? Staying present with these sensations and at some point, your notice your mind wandering away from here, just breathing in and bringing attention back to touching. Exploring as if it was the very first time you were touching this. And noticing all sensations presents with a curious mind. Not trying to force anything happening, not trying to modify your experience in any shape or form, just noticing what is here just as it is.

Now shifting your attention to your sense of smelling. Letting the aroma present in this object being taken in by your nostrils. Not forcing anything, just letting whatever is present here just arrive as it does. Noticing what is pleasant, neutral or unpleasant, without judging it, just experimenting as moments passing through. And smelling again, and noticing with a curious mind what is here that can be smelled, just as it is.

Now bringing gently your attention to the sense of hearing and exploring moment by moment what kind of sounds are present in this object. Noticing your fingers and nails passing over the surface, shaking the object, and noticing sounds just as they are. And as you breathe out letting of all thoughts that may rise in the mind, and simply staying with the sensations as they are.

Now bringing the object and placing it on the tongue. Exploring all tastes, as you slowly chew. Bringing your attention to the felt sensations in the mouth, moment by moment. What sensations are here that you don't usually pay attention to? Exploring all sensations with gentle awareness.

We are now moving towards the end of this practice, so slowly taking your attention away from the felt sensations of digesting and bringing it back to the room. Let's spend a few minutes exploring what you noticed during this experiment."

Following the guided practice the therapist runs an inquiry over what kind of experiences showed up for the patient, and the way to process this information may turn out like this:

Therapist: Tell me what did you notice during this exercise.
Patient: Quite different, I never had eaten a raisin so slowly
Therapist: And as you were slowing down into the experience, what did you notice?
Patient: I felt the texture and I could actually taste the raisin. I was quite surprised, because initially I thought I wouldn't be able to taste just one single raisin.

Therapist: What flavors were there?

Patient: I noticed the taste quite strongly, and it was initially dry in the mouth, and then I noticed it changing as I chewed it…

Therapist: What else did you notice?

Patient: How hard it is to stay present… I noticed my mind wandering off a few times. But then I heard your instructions to come back to sensations, and so I did. I also noticed myself having thoughts about it, of how it looked like a brain… but then I took notice I wasn't feeling the raisin anymore, and so I did what you asked which was to breathe out and let go of that thought.

Therapist: Now bringing your mind back to how you were noticing the object, how do you think this way of paying attention to things is different from the usual way you use your attention?

Patient: Definitely slower. I felt like I slowed down. And I was very keen on exploring and seeing how it was like. It was interesting when you asked to pay attention as if it was the first time, and not to judge, because I noticed it was hard to just feeling without jumping into thoughts about it. And one point I was actually judging the raisin, because I was worried after putting my hand on it for so long, that perhaps it would be weird to place in the mouth. So aside from this, I feel like I was really open and receptive to it. And I don't use pay attention to things with a curious mind as we worked on here. At times I felt like I didn't know nothing about it, and I was really child exploring. On my day to say life I am, often rushing, and trying to get things done.

Therapist: Wow… that's wonderful what you shared with me. I was wondering if you would be able to share with me how you paying attention to things this way, non-judgmentally, patiently, with a curious open mind, might be useful in dealing with the sort of emotional difficulties that you often bring to our therapy sessions?

Patient: Perhaps I can remind myself that I can be gentle with what I am experiencing. And… that perhaps I don't have to be so much afraid of my feelings and the challenging moments I go through. I can see things perhaps more like a child, as opposed to jumping into conclusions and getting lost in negative thoughts.

Therapist: Well, thank you so much for sharing these experiences with me. I was wondering if you would find useful to take this practice to your daily life, and perhaps using one or two activities that you do on your day-to-day life and bringing mindfulness to it.

Patient: I will do that. I think I'd like to actually practice this in my meals. I feel like a I could benefit from not rushing so much these times…."

Body Scan

This is another well-known exercise for developing mindfulness skills. It involves asking patients to lie down, or if there is not enough space in the room, can also be practiced sitting. The main learning therapeutic points of the body scan is to let patients connect with their direct felt sense of the body, and to get to know how the body reacts moment by moment. It is also one of the goals of this practice to learn to direct attention to and away specific body parts. This helps patients learn how to bring purpose to attention. Moreover, the practice invites individuals to deal with mind wandering and chattering from a detached and impersonal manner, and get to develop acceptance of sensations coming and going just as they are. Patients who struggle with emotional stress will find this practice useful in terms of learning to recognize how emotions show up in the body, and how to manage these sensations through allowing and creating space for the to just *be* and *pass*, *be* and *pass*, again and again.

Let's see how a brief body scan practice might look like and understand how therapists can dialogue about experiences that show up for patients during it.

"*Therapist*: I will ask you to go through an exercise with me, a little bit like the exercise we did last week, but this time, instead of bringing mindful awareness to an object, we will be directing this attention to the body still, lying down on this little mat here on the floor. So as you let your body weight fall on the floor, feeling each part just releasing and resting, letting go of the expectations of how things should be like, and just opening up the best you can to the experiences as they are here and now. Focusing on the breath for a little while, noticing all the sensations of the air flowing in, and the air flowing out. Let's stay present with this breathing, resting our attention right on these sensations.

Now let's take the attention to the feet and legs. Let's notice what sensations are showing up in this part of the body, moment by moment. See if it is possible to simply notice sensations as they are. Breathing gently in every sensation present, and staying present. Feel the body sensations as if they were unknown and you were meeting them for the very first time in your life. Notice temperature, if there's tension of softness, if they are heavy or light, and simply notice the sensations as they are. Now the attention slowly leaves the feet and legs, and we move it right into the upper body, including the pelvis, the back, the spine, the front part of the body. The chest and arms. Noticing the sensations that are here. Staying present the best you can. With the breathing holding gently each and every sensation that may arise in this upper region of the body. And if some other experience during this practice calls for your attention, perhaps taking time to notice what is showing up in the moment, instead of ignoring or resisting to it, just acknowledging it gently as an experience passing by. And when you can, bringing attention back to the upper body.

If the mind becomes busy remembering, planning, complaining, or simply chattering in any way or form, just noticing the mind "*being busy*". Breathing in gently, in and around these thoughts, and on the out-breath releasing these thoughts away, patiently letting go, and observing them at a distance, and bringing attention back to what's here and now in the body.

Now bringing attention gently to the arms, and hands, and each of the fingers. Just letting awareness move through each and every sensation present in the arms and hands. Being curious as if each sensation was unique. Not observing sensations as being good nor bad, just exploring what is present with an open curiosity and breathing gently into each sensation. "*Whatever is present in the body, just saying to yourself mentally, I can feel these sensations. It's ok to notice whichever sensations are here*." And so, exploring with the mind of a beginner each moment.

Now leaving the arms, and resting attention into the facial area and the whole head. Noticing pleasant, neutral and also unpleasant sensations in the body, for what they are, passing experiences. And letting go of the thoughts as they arise, breathing in gently, welcoming what is here, breathing out gently letting go of thoughts and releasing each sensation into the ground.

Now to end this practice, notice your full body experience from head to have a sense holding your whole body gently in your awareness, and letting sensations just be as they are. Gently breathing in and out of this whole experience, and at your own time, leaving this practice, and bring your attention back to this room, where we are, me and you."

Now, what experiences showed up for you during the body scan?

Patient: It was interesting because I felt my bones, as if there was no flesh, just bones and emptiness. Every time I breathed there came this sensation of bones. And when you were guiding me in the upper body, I felt everything. My organs came up. But it wasn't bad, it was interesting… And then I slept a little. By this time, it was really pleasant.

Therapist: Right, it seems to be you became quite curious about what was going on in the body, and the experience seemed to change all the time. What else did you notice?

Patient: At some point, during the legs and feet I remember my mind was really busy thinking. I could actually myself getting anxious at this time. But as I was slowly guiding my attention to the sensations and you mention for me to notice the sensations as passing experiences, without trying to resist or judge it, little by little, my experience changed.

Therapist: So, it sounds like at the beginning the thoughts popping into your mind was bringing up unpleasant sensations. And it feels like you just notice this happening and slowly invited your attention back in the body, trusting sensations can change moment after moment.

Patient: That's right. As I noticed my mind wasn't resting, I did struggle a bit trying to control these thoughts, but then this made me body become even tighter and tensed. As you saying to notice sensations as they are, and breathe away the thoughts patiently, I felt rest, and then I started my bones and the sensations of the body more fully. This made me free up my mind I guess."

Conclusion

This chapter demonstrated how Mindfulness-Based Cognitive Therapy (MBCT) can be an effective tool in addressing transdiagnostic psychopathological processes that contribute to the maintenance of psychological distress.

Throughout the discussion, key elements in the development of MBCT were addressed as well as the understanding of the processes through which we can stimulate profound changes in the way individuals coming to therapy could relate to their cognitive, emotional and physical suffering.

Examining critical transdiagnostic processes, it was highlighted the detrimental impact of mindlessness on psychological well-being, emphasizing the importance of mindful living as a way to reducing reactivity and stress symptomatology, enhancing cognitive flexibility and fostering a warm and gentle relation to internal private psychological experiences. The monitoring of discrepancies, cognitive reactivity, cognitive fusion, experiential avoidance, rumination, and worrying were elucidated as pervasive processes across various psychological conditions. Each of these processes, when left unaddressed, can contribute to the perpetuation of distress, reinforcing negative thinking patterns and hindering effective coping mechanisms.

By introducing the fundamental components of MBCT interventions, such as attentional training, mindful noticing, decentering and defusion, recognizing mental habits, and gently relating to bodily sensations, the chapter unveiled the variety of skills in mindfulness-oriented psychotherapy aimed at disrupting these maladaptive processes. Attentional training equips individuals with the ability to deliberately shift focus, while mindful noticing encourages non-judgmental observation of internal experiences. Decentering and defusion empower individuals to disentangle from their thoughts, fostering a less personal perspective and promoting emotional resilience. Recognizing mental habits becomes a powerful tool for interrupting cycles of unhelpful thinking, and gently relating to bodily sensations offers a pathway to understanding the impermanence of emotional distress.

In essence, MBCT stands as useful therapeutic tool, providing individuals with a proactive means to navigate the complexities of mental health care. By addressing the intricate interplay of cognitive and emotional processes, MBCT equips individuals with the tools needed to break free from the cycles of psychological distress, worsened by the tendency to live life in auto-pilot mode, not recognizing when we get stuck in mental habits that could reactivate psychological distress over and over. The integration of mindfulness practices into evidence-based psychological therapies, exemplified by MBCT, not only transforms the way we understand and treat mental health but also holds promise in cultivating a more resilient and mindful society.

References

Akbari, M., Seydavi, M., Hosseini, Z. S., Krafft, J., & Levin, M. E. (2022). Experiential avoidance in depression, anxiety, obsessive-compulsive related, and posttraumatic stress disorders: A comprehensive systematic review and meta-analysis. *Journal of Contextual Behavioral Science, 24*, 65–78.

Aldao, A., Nolen-Hoeksema, S., & Schweizer, S. (2010). Emotion-regulation strategies across psychopathology: A meta-analytic review. *Clinical Psychology Review, 2*, 217–237. https://doi.org/10.1016/j.cpr.2009.11.004. Epub 2009 Nov 20. PMID: 20015584.

Bach, P., & Hayes, S. C. (2002). The use of acceptance and commitment therapy to prevent the rehospitalization of psychotic patients: A randomized controlled trial. *Journal of Consulting and Clinical Psychology, 70*(5), 1129–1139. https://doi.org/10.1037/0022-006X.70.5.1129

Bardeen, J. R. (2015). Short-term pain for long-term gain: The role of experiential avoidance in the relation between anxiety sensitivity and emotional distress. *Journal of Anxiety Disorders, 30*, 113–119. https://doi.org/10.1016/j.janxdis.2014.12.013

Cladder-Micus, M. B., van Aalderen, J., Donders, A. R. T., Spijker, J., Vrijsen, J. N., & Speckens, A. E. M. (2018). Cognitive reactivity as outcome and working mechanism of mindfulness-based cognitive therapy for recurrently depressed patients in remission. *Cognition and Emotion, 32*(2), 371–378. https://doi.org/10.1080/02699931.2017.1285753

Cookson, C., Luzon, O., Newland, J., & Kingston, J. (2019). Examining the role of cognitive fusion and experiential avoidance in predicting anxiety and depression. *Journal of Psychology and Psychotherapy: Theory, Research and Practice*. https://doi.org/10.1111/papt.12233

Crane, R. (2023). *Terapia Cognitiva baseada em Mindfulness: Características Distintivas*. Ed. Sinopsys.

Faustino, B. (2021). Transdiagnostic perspective on psychological inflexibility and emotional dysregulation. *Behavioural and Cognitive Psychotherapy, 49*(2), 233–246. https://doi.org/10.1017/S1352465820000600

Faustino, B., & Vasco, A. B. (2020a). Schematic functioning, interpersonal dysfunctional cycles and cognitive fusion in the complementary paradigmatic perspective: Analysis of a clinical sample. *Journal of Contemporary Psychotherapy, 1*, 47–55. https://doi.org/10.1007/s10879-019-09422-x

Faustino, B., & Vasco, A. B. (2020b). Early maladaptive schemas and cognitive fusion on the regulation of psychological needs. *Journal of Contemporary Psychotherapy, 1*, 105–112. https://doi.org/10.1007/s10879-019-09446-3

Faustino, B., Vasco, A. B., Oliveira, J., Lopes, P., & Fonseca, I. (2019). Metacognitive self-assessment scale: Psychometric properties and clinical applications. *Applied Neuropsychology: Adult*. https://doi.org/10.1080/23279095.2019.1671843

Faustino, B., Vasco, A. B., Farinha-Fernandes, A., et al. (2023). Psychological inflexibility as a transdiagnostic construct: Relationships between cognitive fusion, psychological well-being and symptomatology. *Current Psychology, 42*, 6056–6061. https://doi.org/10.1007/s12144-021-01943-w

Friary, V. (2018). *Mindfulness para Crianças: Estratégias da terapia cognitiva baseada em mindfulness*. Ed. Sinopsys.

Hayes, S. C., Wilson, K. G., Gifford, E. V., Follette, V. M., & Strosahl, K. (1996). Experiential avoidance and behavioral disorders: A functional dimensional approach to diagnosis and treatment. *Journal of Consulting and Clinical Psychology, 64*(6), 1152. https://doi.org/10.1037/0022-006X.64.6.1152

Hayes, S. C., Strosahl, K. D., & Wilson, K. G. (2011). *Acceptance and commitment therapy: The process and practice of mindful change* (2nd ed.). The Guilford Press.

Hayes, S. C., Pistorello, J., & Levin, M. E. (2012). Acceptance and commitment therapy as a unified model of behavior change. *The Counseling Psychologist, 40*(7), 976–1002. https://doi.org/10.1177/0011000012460836

Higgins, E. T. (1987). Self-discrepancy: A theory relating self and affect. *Psychological Review, 94*(3), 319–340. https://doi.org/10.1037/0033-295X.94.3.319

Linehan, M. M., Schmidt, H. I., Dimeff, L. A., Craft, J. C., Katner, J., & Comtois, K. A. (1999). Dialectical behavior therapy for patients with borderline personality disorder and drug-dependence. *American Journal on Addiction, 8*, 279–292.

Lynch, T. R., Morse, J. Q., Mendelson, T., & Robins, C. J. (2003). Dialectical behavior therapy for depressed older adults: A randomized pilot study. *American Journal of Geriatric Psychiatry, 11*, 33–45. https://doi.org/10.1097/00019442-200301000-00006

Nolen-Hoeksema, S., Wisco, B. E., & Lyubomirsky, S. (2008). Rethinking rumination. *Perspectives on Psychological Science, 3*, 400–424.

Ruiz, F. J. (2010). A review of acceptance and commitment therapy (ACT) empirical evidence: Correlational, experimental psychopathology, component and outcome studies. *Revista Internacional de Psicología y Terapia Psicológica, 10*, 125–162.

Spinhoven, P., Drost, J., de Rooij, M., van Hemert, A. M., & Penninx, B. W. (2014). A longitudinal study of experiential avoidance in emotional disorders. *Behavior Therapy, 45*, 840–850. https://doi.org/10.1016/j.beth.2014.07.001

Watkins, E., & Roberts, H. (2020). Reflecting on rumination: Consequences, causes, mechanisms and treatment of rumination. *Behavior Research and Therapy, 127*, Article number 103573.

Chapter 6
Dialectical Behavior Therapy (DBT)

Wilson Vieira Melo, Ramiro Figueiredo Catelan, Lucianne Jobim Valdivia, and Jan Luiz Leonardi

Introduction

Dialectical Behavior Therapy (DBT) is a psychosocial treatment developed during the 1980s by the American psychologist Marsha M. Linehan, originally aiming at treating women with high levels of suicidal behavior (Linehan, 1993). Linehan observed that the conventional therapeutic approaches at the time often fell short in effectively treating individuals with intense psychological suffering. Traditional cognitive-behavioral therapy (CBT), for instance, emphasized change and problem-solving, which could sometimes be perceived as invalidating by the clients, leading to increased resistance and emotional distress. To counter this, she integrated the dialectical philosophy, which emphasizes the synthesis of opposites, balancing the need for change with the need for acceptance. This approach involves acknowledging and validating clients' experiences while still advocating for change and improvement (Koerner, 2012).

Over time, DBT became the most robust evidence-based treatment for borderline personality disorder (BPD). Its creation was largely influenced by Linehan's own struggles with a BPD personal diagnosis and her professional experiences in treating individuals with severe emotion dysregulation and suicidal behaviors. People with BPD may exhibit numerous ineffective patterns in cognitive, emotional, behavioral, and interpersonal spheres. DBT presents an organized and systematic approach, where a team of psychologists shares foundational beliefs about the treatment and the client. Individuals with drastic BPD symptoms often resort to suicide attempts as a means to alleviate their suffering or due to intense impulsivity traits.

W. V. Melo (✉) · R. F. Catelan · L. J. Valdivia
Porto Alegre, RS, Brazil

J. L. Leonardi
Catanduva, SP, Brazil

A. C. Ornelas (ed.), *Transdiagnostic Approaches in Cognitive Behavioral Therapy*, https://doi.org/10.1007/978-3-031-63494-9_6

DBT views suicidal behaviors, for instance, as maladaptive problem-solving strategies and employs well-researched and empirically validated techniques to assist clients in resolving their life issues more adaptively and skillfully (Pederson, 2015).

Biosocial Model

The biosocial model proposes that a history of interaction between biological vulnerability and a chronically invalidating environment can create and maintain the behavioral, cognitive, and emotional patterns observed in individuals with pervasive emotion dysregulation (Linehan, 1993). In this context, three key concepts are essential to understand the biopsychosocial model: emotion dysregulation, biological vulnerability, and invalidation.

Emotion dysregulation is primarily characterized by five factors: (1) increased susceptibility to experiencing emotions intensely; (2) difficulty in inhibiting impulsive behaviors related to intense emotions; (3) difficulty in reducing physiological activation involved in the emotional episode; (4) difficulty in acting in accordance with one's goals and values when such action differs from the behavioral inclination evoked by the emotion; and (5) difficulty in focusing on anything other than the event that triggered the emotion (Linehan, 2015). Pervasive emotion dysregulation is the inability to regulate emotions across a wide range of situations, i.e., a global pattern of emotion dysregulation that can lead to various problematic behaviors, such as suicide, self-harm, and substance abuse (Koerner, 2012).

Biological vulnerability is characterized by three elements: (1) high sensitivity to stimuli, meaning the individual reacts to low-threshold emotional triggers; (2) high reactivity, i.e., the individual experiences and expresses emotions extremely intensely; and (3) slow return to baseline, indicating that the emotional experience persists for a long time. Biological vulnerability can be essentially genetic (the individual is born more susceptible) and/or include environmental factors, such as traumatic experiences that affect brain development and functioning (Koerner, 2012; Linehan, 2015).

The chronic invalidating environment involves the punishment or suppression of an individual's expressions about their private experiences (feelings, sensations, and thoughts). Emotional expression is judged as inappropriate, wrong, or pathological; it is minimized, ridiculed, or not taken seriously; it is ignored or neglected. Typical examples of invalidation include statements like: "You have no reason to feel that way"; "Stop crying or I'll give you a real reason to cry"; "If you really wanted to, you could do it". In such a context, the learning to describe private events is impaired, and feeling itself becomes aversive, leading the individual to try to escape or avoid their emotional reactions, to invalidate what they feel, think, and do, and, consequently, to seek from others the "correct" way to feel, think, and act. Furthermore, as an invalidating environment typically does not teach emotional regulation and reacts favorably only to intense emotional demonstrations (i.e., reinforces only extreme behaviors), the individual escalates their expressions. For example, instead of once again stating they are suffering, which was invalidated, they may resort to self-harm, which garners validation, care, attention, etc.; when self-harm ceases to produce the same effect, they may threaten suicide; eventually, they may attempt suicide. Together, the invalidation of usual emotional expressions, the consequent development of a "phobia" of one's own emotions, and the intermittent reinforcement of severe manifestations produce a fluctuation between emotional inhibition and emotional "explosion," both fraught with much suffering. To worsen matters, a typical invalidating environment simplifies the individual's difficulties and thus does not teach problem-solving skills, making failure more likely, leading to more invalidation (Koerner, 2012).

Koerner (2012) states that the existence of emotion dysregulation may have more genetic or more environmental origins. Thus, for individuals born with a high degree of biological vulnerability, an invalidating environment that might not affect others can lead to pervasive emotion dysregulation. Conversely, individuals who are genetically less vulnerable might develop pervasive emotion dysregulation due to a severe chronic invalidating environment.

In conclusion, pervasive emotion dysregulation originates from the interaction between two factors—biological vulnerability and an invalidating environment. Although the biopsychosocial model was originally developed as a theoretical proposal to understand the etiology of borderline personality disorder, it has also been used as an explanatory model for emotion dysregulation present in other psychiatric disorders (Koerner, 2012). This model underscores the complexity of emotion dysregulation, highlighting the interplay of genetic predispositions and environmental factors. It suggests that both biological and environmental influences are crucial in understanding and addressing emotion dysregulation in various psychiatric conditions.

Treatment Modes

DBT is a multimodal intervention that consists of different components as part of its standard treatment: individual psychotherapy, skills training group, phone coaching, and a therapist consultation team. One can only say they are treating a client in a standard DBT procedure if the four modes are being fully applied. There is a final component related to ancillary treatments. We'll delve deeper into each of these in the following sections of this chapter.

Individual Therapy

As previously mentioned, DBT is unique in its multi-modal approach, comprising four components: individual therapy, skills training group, phone coaching, and therapist consultation team. Each mode plays a crucial role in the treatment process, with individual therapy being a cornerstone. A typical DBT individual therapy session occurs once a week and lasts between 45 and 60 min. The individual therapist is responsible for providing guidance and coordination for the client's treatment (Koerner, 2012).

DBT's individual therapy sessions are, at the same time, highly structured and flexible. They usually begin with greeting the client, noting their actual emotional state, and engaging them in mindfulness exercises to prepare for the session's work. The therapist then reviews other aspects of the client's treatment, including progress in skills groups and recent appointments with other providers. The diary card, a tool that must be completed daily by the client, is reviewed to identify treatment targets and set the agenda for the session. This review includes validation, support, and encouragement from the therapist. The main work of the session then focuses on addressing these targets with appropriate strategies (not only with DBT skills, but also with other solutions, such as cognitive modification, exposure, and contingency management) (Pederson, 2015).

The main tasks of the individual therapy include:

1. Building and maintaining a therapeutic relationship: The therapist must create a safe, accepting, and empathetic environment. This relationship is based on trust, validation, and an understanding that the therapist and client are working collaboratively. It's essential for the therapist to balance acceptance and change strategies, showing genuine compassion while also pushing the client towards growth and change.
2. Conducting behavioral analyses: A critical task for the DBT individual therapist is to conduct thorough behavioral chain analyses, particularly of problematic behaviors such as self-harm, suicidal ideation, and therapy-interfering behaviors. A chain analysis allows both therapist and client to understand the sequence of events, thoughts, emotions, and actions that lead to these behaviors, which is essential to help the client to reduce and eliminate target behaviors and develop more effective coping strategies.
3. Targeting and prioritizing treatment goals: In DBT, treatment goals are hierarchical. The highest priority is given to life-threatening behaviors, followed by therapy-interfering behaviors, and then by behaviors that significantly impair the client's quality of life. The therapist must adeptly identify and prioritize these targets in each session, ensuring that the most critical issues are addressed first.
4. Skills training and generalization: While skills training is often conducted in a group setting, the individual therapist has the crucial task of helping the client apply these skills to specific challenges in their daily life. This involves integrating skills into various contexts and ensuring that the client understands and can use these skills effectively when needed. The therapist aids in troubleshooting problems in skill application and reinforces the client's progress in learning and using these skills. The therapist is also responsible for teaching the client skills that they might urgently need and have not been addressed in the skills training classes yet.

5. Managing crisis situations: a DBT individual therapist is often called upon to assist in crisis situations, particularly when clients are at risk of engaging in life-threatening behavior. They must be skilled in crisis intervention techniques, helping the clients to de-escalate emotions, apply distress tolerance skills, and return to a safer state of mind.
6. Promoting motivation and addressing therapy-interfering behaviors: Keeping clients motivated and engaged in therapy is a significant part of the DBT individual therapist's role. This includes addressing any behaviors that might interfere with the client's participation in therapy, such as missing sessions, being unresponsive in sessions, or not completing homework. The therapist works with the client to overcome these challenges and stay committed to the treatment process.

Skills Training Group

DBT recognizes that many of the challenges faced by individuals with emotion dysregulation stem largely from a lack of learning skills to cope with intense emotional activation. Learning and systematically applying problem-solving and avoiding maladaptive responses are among the primary goals of DBT. During the development of this approach, Linehan stated that individual therapy wasn't enough to address the clients' need for learning new skills, and then created a specific treatment mode for that purpose, the skills training group.

One of the initial steps in skills training is to demonstrate, within the client's context, that the way they have been responding to problematic situations is not effective. Therefore, the chain analysis of current behaviors, their consequences, and providing alternative solutions are crucial to engage the client in learning new skills. It is not uncommon for clients to be familiar with some of the taught skills; however, they may not know how to use them effectively, resulting in ineffective actions.

According to Linehan (1993), the skills learning process involves three phases: (1) skill acquisition; (2) skill strengthening; and (3) skill generalization. In the skill acquisition phase, skills are taught in a didactic manner and modeled, especially within the therapeutic relationship. During the skill strengthening phase, the client is encouraged to use the acquired skills in role-plays with the therapist in simulated situations both inside and outside of therapy (behavioral rehearsal). In these situations, the therapist's reinforcement and feedback are crucial for the consolidation of learning. The generalization phase is where the client learns to apply the skills flexibly and adapted to the context, engaging in tasks between sessions with the therapist's guidance to assist in using the skills in real-life problem situations.

Currently, skills training within or outside standard DBT (comprising skills training, individual psychotherapy, telephone coaching, and a therapist consultation team) has proven to be an effective intervention for improving difficulties in emotional regulation. This is not limited to borderline personality disorder but extends to individuals with various diagnoses (Durpoix et al., 2023), whether used as a standalone intervention or not (Lyng et al., 2020; Warner & Murphy, 2022).

Regarding the delivery format of the intervention, skills training can be provided to clients undergoing individual psychotherapy within the DBT approach, as well as those following other theoretical approaches. Another consideration is the increasing trend of skills training groups taking place online rather than exclusively face-to-face. In 2021, van Leeuwen et al. conducted a review on the efficacy of online DBT, noting the scarcity of studies in this area and the heterogeneity of results from interventions conducted thus far. Consequently, they state that there is insufficient evidence to prefer online skills training when in-person options are available.

The organization and structure of skills training groups require two therapists with distinct and well-defined roles. The group leader is responsible for teaching the skills objectively and didactically. The co-leader serves as an assistant teacher, providing more direct assistance to each group member and managing tensions arising from interactions among participants.

The presence of two leaders in each group is necessary given that managing situations among participants with high emotion dysregulation can be extremely challenging. It is not uncommon for participants to become emotionally activated during sessions and may act impulsively or even experience crises. In these moments, it is the leaders' responsibility to organize a safe environment and use dialectical skills and strategies to handle the situation, providing the necessary assistance for the participant to regain composure.

During the initial individual interviews for participant admission, which marks the beginning of the therapeutic alliance, an assessment is conducted to determine the relevance of their inclusion in the group. Participants are also informed about the objectives and functioning of the training. It is recommended that, in pre-group meetings, each participant fills out a form containing, among other pertinent information, the contact details of individuals to be reached in case of a crisis.

The first group sessions serve to integrate participants, familiarize them with the DBT assumptions, establish agreements on group behavior and relationships, and define training objectives. Among the group agreements, it can be established that there will be direct communication between skills trainers and the individual therapist of each participant, especially to report any situations that occurred in the sessions that deserve attention in psychotherapy. In this sense, it is agreed that, in case of a crisis, the participant should seek help from their individual psychotherapist and not the skills trainer (unless the therapist is also the trainer).

Training in skills can be structured in different ways according to the levels of intervention (prevention and/or treatment), target audience, and schedule. There are fundamental skills to be taught that are considered essential within a program focused on individuals with typical behaviors of high emotion dysregulation (i.e., emotional crises, self-harming behaviors). However, it is possible to customize the training according to the audience and the emphasis intended for the target audience (substance use, communication and sociability skills, compulsive eating, etc.), and the therapist's skills manual (Linehan, 2015) provides examples of previously tested schedules with various audiences and durations.

In addition to the initial sheets of general guidelines, there are four sets of skills that can be taught during the training in a modular format: (1) mindfulness; (2) distress tolerance; (3) emotional regulation; and (4) interpersonal effectiveness. Mindfulness skills are central to the skills training because they are necessary for the participant to develop awareness of their behaviors, impulses, functioning, and to choose wisely (wise mind) and equanimously (middle path) how to deal with external and internal adverse situations. Learning to observe one thing at a time, describing without judgment, participating in the experience being lived in the present moment provides the necessary conditions for us to act effectively in each situation, considering what we intend and what is important to us.

The second set of skills is distress tolerance, which aims to teach new ways to "survive" moments of crisis. Crises are understood in this module as moments of high emotional activation in response to external situations or even triggered by internal factors such as mood swings, for example. Learning how to tolerate and "get through" difficult moments without making them worse is crucial for the emotional regulation process. In this module, skills for accepting reality are also presented. Many of the crises experienced by clients may arise from facing aversive situations that generate reactions of outrage and non-acceptance. Facing reality as it is presented, without rejecting it, is the first step in changing how we will effectively deal with it.

Emotional regulation is the third set of skills in which, initially, "emotional literacy" is provided. Understanding emotions, how and why they arise, and their functions help the participant better understand their own emotional functioning without invalidating or judging themselves. Throughout the module, strategies are offered on how to modify emotional responses that are automatically triggered, both in their content and intensity, as well as strategies to reduce vulnerability. Participants are invited to guide their actions by important values to be developed within what each one understands as a valuable life.

Interpersonal effectiveness is the fourth module and is organized to address factors that interfere with interpersonal effectiveness, such as obtaining goals skillfully and developing abilities to navigate the middle path. Learning how to communicate effectively, articulate arguments, and have a clear understanding of what one wants to communicate are fundamental skills to be acquired and developed when living in society. Individuals with high emotion dysregulation often struggle to create and maintain healthy relationships or find themselves in harmful relationships. Therefore, the training covers a series of strategies to assist individuals in building healthy relationships and recognizing and ultimately ending destructive relationships.

As previously discussed, in DBT, there is a dialectical balance between acceptance and change, and the skills taught stem from this balance. The training aims to develop skills that will assist the client in understanding and coping with their traits and adversities. This includes learning to accept them and improving the ability to handle such situations, while also addressing skills focused on problem-solving and behavioral change.

Phone Coaching

The phone coaching is envisioned as one of the treatment modalities within standard DBT, with specific objectives and structure. The primary goal of telephone contact is to assist the client in applying and generalizing the skills learned in therapy when problematic situations arise. This contact provides extra time for the client and therapist to address crises, thereby preventing potential suicidal and parasuicidal behaviors.

The therapist must make it clear that, in a crisis where the client is unable to cope, they can make a phone call. In such cases, the therapist will assist the client in managing the current crisis, but not all factors surrounding the situation will be addressed. In other words, it is not a full consultation; only crisis management will be provided.

If the client calls the therapist after engaging in problematic behavior, the 24-h rule will be applied. This rule stipulates that the client will not be able to call the therapist within the subsequent 24 h after engaging in parasuicidal behavior, considering that there is no longer a need for therapist assistance, as the client has already "resolved the problem." Establishing this rule in advance aims to reinforce that the client should contact the therapist before engaging in problematic behavior to prevent it and reinforce alternative ways of dealing with the crisis.

Teaching the client how to ask for help is also one of the objectives of telephone coaching. Learning how to effectively seek help from others is crucial for individuals who, due to a lack of skills, may struggle to do so in an organized manner or may not ask for help at all. Some people may find it challenging to contact the therapist in advance, and planning phone calls between the two can be a combined task to address this situation. This task models how the client seeks help, reinforcing their skills when relying on their support network.

When making a phone call, the therapist needs to keep two main directions in mind: being mindful and focusing on skills. As mentioned earlier, phone calls are not intended to provide therapy but rather to manage crises. Tasks during a phone contact to handle a crisis include assessing imminent risk, removing the client from means available for problematic behavior, quantifying the level of distress, and using the previously developed crisis plan.

Therapists often wonder about the possibility of excessive phone calls from clients, and this can occur. In such cases, this situation should be addressed as a behavior that interferes with therapy since it may overload the therapist and, consequently, the therapeutic relationship. Additionally, it may not help the client develop skills and autonomy to manage their own crises, potentially leading to dependency.

Consultation Team

The consultation team plays a vital role in the overall effectiveness and integrity of a DBT program, to the point that one cannot say they are a DBT therapist according to the standard model if they are not a part of a consultation team. DBT is a complex, demanding psychosocial treatment, both for clients and therapists, and the consultation team serves as a crucial support system for therapists. This group, often composed of other trained DBT therapists, provides a unique platform for professional development, support, and maintaining the fidelity of the DBT model (Koerner, 2012).

A DBT consultation team meeting is structured to foster collaboration and support among therapists, adhering to specific guidelines to maximize its effectiveness. Typically, these meetings are held weekly, underscoring their importance in maintaining the therapists' adherence to DBT principles and providing consistent support. The meetings usually start with a mindfulness exercise, which serves to center the team members and prepare them for the work ahead. The main body of the meeting is devoted to case consultation, where therapists present challenging cases and receive feedback and guidance from their peers. This process is not just about problem-solving but also involves mutual support, enhancing skills, and ensuring adherence to DBT protocols. The team also discusses administrative and training issues, ensuring that all members are current with DBT methodology and practices. Importantly, these meetings provide a space for therapists to express their own vulnerabilities and seek support, which is critical in a treatment as demanding as DBT. The regularity and structure of these meetings are fundamental in maintaining the quality and integrity of the therapeutic approach (Pederson, 2015).

The main tasks of the consultation team include:

1. Treating the therapist: the primary function of a DBT consultation team is to provide support for the therapists, as it is acknowledged that treating challenging and complex clients with severe psychological suffering can be often demanding and exhaustive. The team acts as a therapeutic entity for therapists themselves, aiming at mitigating therapists' burnout and providing a supportive and collaborative environment where they can address their own challenges, vulnerabilities, and growth areas. In the demanding realm of treating clients with severe emotion dysregulation, therapists are at risk of burnout, compassion fatigue, and secondary traumatic stress. The consultation team offers a platform where therapists can openly discuss their emotional responses, ethical dilemmas, and personal triggers related to their work. This process not only helps in reducing the emotional toll on therapists but also enhances their therapeutic skills, as they receive feedback, guidance, and validation from their peers. The team helps therapists maintain their objectivity, prevent over-identification with clients, and uphold the therapeutic boundaries, which are critical for effective treatment delivery. Moreover, it reinforces adherence to the DBT framework, ensuring that therapists do not deviate from the model under emotional strain. By focusing on the well-being and professional development of the therapist, the DBT

consultation team indirectly improves the quality of care provided to clients, as a well-supported therapist is more likely to be effective, empathetic, and resilient in their clinical work.

2. Skill development for therapists: The team facilitates continuous learning and skill development. DBT is a skills-based therapy, and the consultation team helps therapists refining their use of these skills, learning new techniques, and staying updated on the latest research and developments in the field. DBT consultation team serves as a dynamic learning environment where therapists enhance their clinical skills and deepen their understanding of DBT principles. Through regular meetings, team members engage in discussions, role-plays, and review of therapy sessions, which facilitate the honing of specific DBT skills such as mindfulness, distress tolerance, emotion regulation, and interpersonal effectiveness. This collaborative setting allows therapists to learn from each other's experiences and insights, fostering a culture of continuous improvement and professional growth. The consultation team also addresses the challenges therapists face in applying these skills in diverse and complex clinical scenarios, offering practical solutions and alternative approaches. This ongoing skills development is crucial not only for adhering to the rigorous standards of DBT but also for adapting and evolving the treatment to meet the unique needs of each client. By regularly participating in these skill-building exercises, therapists maintain a high level of competence and confidence in their practice, directly benefiting the therapeutic process and outcomes for their clients.
3. Maintaining fidelity to the DBT model: The consultation team also must ensure that the treatment provided adheres to the DBT model's principles and procedures. DBT is a structured psychosocial program with a series of specific components. The consultation team helps therapists adhere to these methods, ensuring that they are not deviating from the model or integrating incompatible techniques. This is important for the effectiveness of DBT, as the treatment's success is partly attributed to its structured, evidence-based approach. The team regularly reviews cases, discusses treatment plans, and provides feedback, which helps in maintaining the integrity of the DBT model. By doing so, the team ensures that clients receive the best possible treatment, which is crucial for their recovery.
4. Enhancing therapeutic skills and managing challenging cases: Finally, the consultation team aids therapists in enhancing their therapeutic skills, especially in managing challenging cases. DBT clients often present complex and severe psychological issues, making their treatment challenging. The consultation team allows therapists to discuss these challenging cases in a confidential and supportive environment. Through discussion, role-playing, and feedback, therapists can develop more effective strategies for handling difficult situations. This collaborative problem-solving approach is invaluable, as it provides therapists with a broader range of perspectives and solutions. Moreover, the team encourages therapists to practice self-reflection and self-care, which are crucial for their well-being and effectiveness as clinicians.

In summary, the consultation team in DBT is essential for supporting therapists, preventing and reducing their burnout, ensuring adherence to the DBT model, and enhancing therapeutic skills, especially in challenging cases. This team provides a vital support system that underpins the success and sustainability of DBT as a therapeutic approach.

Ancillary Treatment

The ancillary treatments encompass all other professionals who are also crucial in treatment but do not participate in the consultation team meetings. These professionals may be part of the inpatient team when the client is admitted to a hospital or psychiatric clinic, for example. Additionally, professionals like psychopharmacologists and other medical specialties may be included in the list of ancillary treatments when they are not part of the consultation team. Other professionals such as nutritionists, physical educators, vocational counselors, speech therapists, nurses etc., can also be mentioned in this category.

This fifth component of treatment is the only one that may not necessarily be present because many individuals receiving DBT treatment may not require all of these additional services. The inclusion of these auxiliary treatments depends on the specific needs of the individual undergoing DBT.

Primary Targets

The primary targets of DBT include specific areas of intervention that are prioritized initially. The main goal of treatment at the outset is to address behaviors that pose a risk to life. These behaviors encompass suicidal actions as well as homicidal tendencies. Moreover, behaviors that directly interfere with the client's ability to engage in therapy are also identified as primary targets. Lastly, behaviors that significantly impact overall quality of life are listed as primary targets for interventions in DBT. Let's delve deeper into each of these three subcategories of primary treatment targets.

Life Threatening Behaviors

Target behaviors are divided into four stages in DBT. In the first stage, which is the highest in the treatment hierarchy, is focused on addressing behaviors that pose a direct risk to the client's life. This stage prioritizes the treatment of life-threatening actions, which include suicidal behaviors, self-harm, and suicidal ideation.

Suicidal actions refer to any behaviors where the individual attempts to end their own life. These can range from well-planned attempts to more impulsive actions. It's crucial for DBT to address these behaviors immediately, as they pose the most immediate risk to the client's life. Some examples of behaviors that put one's own life at risk include: hanging oneself; shooting oneself with a firearm; jumping from high places; consuming poison; setting oneself on fire; ingesting a large quantity of medication; using cocaine with ambivalence about the possibility of death by overdose (even without noticeable suicidal intent), consuming a substance with the intention of causing bodily harm (e.g., drinking with liver disease to further damage the liver); among others.

Self-harm, the next focus of Stage 1, includes any form of self-injury that a person engages in without the intent to die, but as a way of coping with overwhelming emotions. This can manifest in various forms, such as cutting, burning, or other means of inflicting physical harm on oneself. The intention behind self-harm is often to relieve emotional pain or distress, rather than to end one's life, but it's a dangerous behavior that can lead to severe physical injuries and sets a harmful pattern that needs urgent attention.

Suicidal ideation encompasses thoughts, fantasies, or preoccupations with ending one's own life. While not every person who experiences suicidal thoughts will act on them, they are a significant risk factor for both suicide attempts and completed suicide.

Therapy-Interfering Behaviors

The second category in the target hierarchy concerns therapy-interfering behaviors (TIBs), which are any behaviors recognized as significant obstacles to the effectiveness of treatment, leading them to be addressed with high priority if life-threatening behaviors are not present or have already been addressed. TIBs can arise from both the client and the therapist, and managing these behaviors is crucial for the progress and success of the treatment (Chapman & Rosenthal, 2016).

From the client's perspective, TIBs include a range of actions or inactions that hinder the therapeutic process or the client's progress in therapy. These behaviors can be varied, such as missing or arriving late to therapy sessions, not completing homework assignments, being non-collaborative or hostile in sessions, and resisting engaging in the therapeutic work. TIBs also encompass behaviors that directly challenge the therapeutic alliance, such as not being honest with the therapist, minimizing or exaggerating symptoms, or not applying learned skills outside of therapy. In DBT, these behaviors are seen not as character flaws or willful defiance but as part of the client's struggle with emotional regulation or as learned behaviors stemming from past experiences. Addressing these behaviors involves the therapist and client collaboratively identifying and understanding the factors contributing to the TIBs and using DBT strategies to modify them. This process is essential for creating a more effective therapeutic environment and for the client's overall progress in therapy (Van Dijk, 2013).

TIBs can also originate from the therapists themselves, impacting the treatment's efficacy. These behaviors may include being judgmental, lacking empathy, responding in a non-validated manner, or having difficulty managing boundaries. Therapists might also inadvertently reinforce unhelpful client behaviors or fail to adhere strictly to the DBT model, which can disrupt the therapy process. In DBT, therapist TIBs are addressed through the consultation team, where therapists receive support and constructive feedback from their peers. The team acts as a platform for therapists to reflect on their own behaviors, receive guidance on adhering to DBT principles, and improve their therapeutic skills. This aspect of addressing therapist TIBs is crucial, as it not only enhances the therapist's effectiveness but also models the process of self-reflection and change for the client (Pederson, 2015).

The management of TIBs in DBT involves a balance of acceptance and change strategies. Therapists use validation to acknowledge the client's feelings and experiences that might be driving their TIBs, while simultaneously using problem-solving and other behavioral strategies to change these behaviors. This approach helps clients feel understood and supported, while also empowering them to take responsibility for their actions and their therapy process. The use of diary cards and chain analyses also provides a structured way to track and address TIBs, helping both the client and therapist to understand the triggers and consequences of these behaviors. Through this process, TIBs are not just reduced, but are replaced with more effective behaviors that support the client's therapeutic goals and general well-being (Chapman & Rosenthal, 2016).

Essentially, TIBs are a critical focus in DBT, acknowledging that both client and therapist can contribute to these behaviors. Addressing TIBs involves a nuanced understanding of their origins and a collaborative effort to modify them, supported by the structured strategies of DBT and the reflective practice provided by the consultation team. This comprehensive approach ensures that both clients and therapists are working effectively towards the goals of therapy.

Quality of Life Interfering Behaviors

Of the primary targets in treatment in DBT, we have those behaviors that directly interfere with the individual's quality of life, which can often be diverse. Among such behaviors, we can mention those related to psychiatric comorbidities with other disorders. For example, a client presenting behaviors related to panic disorder, obsessive-compulsive disorder, bipolar disorder, and attention deficit/hyperactivity disorder will have their symptoms addressed as a primary target of treatment.

Among the primary targets, we should prioritize behaviors that first pose a risk to life, and secondly, those that pose a risk to therapy. In that way, we will have a clear hierarchy regarding what should be prioritized in the intervention. Thus, it makes complete sense to have a transdiagnostic treatment in DBT, since the interventions will not be focused on specific syndromes but rather on those targets considered primary within the theory.

We can also include as behaviors that interfere with quality-of-life other illnesses, such as obesity, diabetes, gastric reflux, asthma, etc. Difficulties and other interpersonal relationship problems, issues with the legal system, with work/school, or even housing. There are numerous situations that will be considered a threat to the individual's quality of life, and all of these will be addressed within this hierarchy of targets.

In conclusion, we can understand that DBT is not a protocol-driven treatment but rather a principle-guided treatment. Therefore, the hierarchy of targets makes it clear what the priority of intervention is, even in cases where various demands compete for the therapist's attention.

Conclusion

DBT is the treatment of first choice for clients diagnosed with severe BPD and is one of the most well-studied and structured approaches for treating complex cases. However, using evidence-based treatment approaches outside of a research context is not simply "plug and play". Some questions are important to guide the clinician's work, including deciding whether the best strategy for each particular case will be to adopt or adapt the previously tested model.

Some implications to consider involve the fact that some modifications may or may not work as well as the original model. Evidence-based therapy protocols have a high level of methodological control for intervention, including a treatment structure that often cannot be reproduced in an ecological context, meaning the real world. Furthermore, in research settings, offering a different model from the one already tested may bring complications regarding ethical aspects.

It's important to keep in mind some points that can help resolve this dilemma between adopting or adapting the original treatment model. The first issue is to radically accept the dialectical tension between the two poles and seek synthesis. Secondly, it's essential to clearly identify whether the plan to be followed is to adopt or adapt the already tested model. In cases where the treatment model will be employed for the first time in a mental health service, it's best to start with a small, firmly focused pilot program. It's important to consider typical issues in your reality, functional and operational problems, as well as issues related to treatment non-adherence. Finally, it's indispensable to use all available scientific literature to increase the chances of success. DBT is a great model treatment and we hardly invite you to know more about this approach.

References

Chapman, A. L., & Rosenthal, M. Z. (2016). *Managing therapy-interfering behavior: Strategies from dialectical behavior therapy*. American Psychological Association.

Durpoix, A., Lachaux, E., Weiner, L., & Weibel, S. (2023, December 21). Transdiagnostic skills training group of dialectical behavior therapy: A long-term naturalistic study. *Borderline Personal Disorder Emotion Dysregulation, 10*(1), 37. PMID: 38124187; PMCID: PMC10734074. https://doi.org/10.1186/s40479-023-00243-y.

Koerner, K. (2012). *Doing dialectical behavior therapy: A practical guide*. Guilford Press.

Linehan, M. M. (1993). *Cognitive-behavioral treatment of borderline personality disorder*. Guilford Press.

Linehan, M. M. (2015). *DBT skills training handouts and worksheets*. Guilford Press.

Lyng, J., Swales, M. A., Hastings, R. P., Millar, T., Duffy, D. J., & Booth, R. (2020, February). Standalone DBT group skills training versus standard (i.e. all modes) DBT for borderline personality disorder: A natural quasi-experiment in routine clinical practice. *Community Mental Health Journal, 56*(2), 238–250. Epub 2019 Oct 31. PMID: 31673877. https://doi.org/10.1007/s10597-019-00485-7.

Pederson, L. D. (2015). *Dialectical behavior therapy: A contemporary guide for practitioners*. Wiley.

Van Dijk, S. (2013). *DBT made simple: A step-by-step guide to dialectical behavior therapy*. New Harbinger Publications.

Van Leeuwen, H., Sinnaeve, R., Witteveen, U., Van Daele, T., Ossewaarde, L., Egger, J. I. M., & van den Bosch, L.M.C. (2021, October 30). Reviewing the availability, efficacy and clinical utility of Telepsychology in dialectical behavior therapy (Tele-DBT). *Borderline Personality Disorder and Emotion Dysregulation, 8*(1), 26. PMID: 34717772; PMCID: PMC8556811. https://doi.org/10.1186/s40479-021-00165-7.

Warner, N., & Murphy, M. (2022, February). Dialectical behaviour therapy skills training for individuals with substance use disorder: A systematic review. *Drug and Alcohol Review, 41*(2), 501–516. Epub 2021 Aug 1. PMID: 34337811. https://doi.org/10.1111/dar.13362.

Chapter 7
Widening the Reach of Cognitive Therapy with Trial-Based Cognitive Therapy Techniques

Irismar Reis de Oliveira

Introduction

Trial-Based Cognitive Therapy (TBCT) represents an innovative therapeutic approach that has emerged in the last two decades, inspired by Franz Kafka's seminal novel, "The Trial" (Kafka, 1925/1998). This approach draws parallels with the existential and accusatory narrative in Kafka's work, where the protagonist faces a relentless trial based on unknown charges. Similarly, in TBCT, patients confront their self-imposed trials, where they are both the accused and the accuser, based on their core beliefs (CBs). Under the guidance of therapists, patients engage in a structured process akin to a court trial to examine, challenge, and reframe these ingrained beliefs. This method not only mirrors the internal conflict experienced by many but also resonates with the themes in Kafka's narrative, reflecting an endless and opaque struggle against an undefined accusation (de Oliveira, 2011).

TBCT is rooted in the principles of cognitive-behavioral therapy (CBT), particularly those developed by Aaron Beck (1976), but it extends these principles by incorporating techniques from various therapeutic models, such as Gestalt therapy (notably the empty chair technique), compassion-focused therapy, metacognitive therapy, mindfulness, and relational models (de Oliveira, 2016). This approach is transdiagnostic, manualized, and features its own unique case conceptualization, emphasizing the modification of patients' CBs, especially those that are self-directed (de Oliveira, 2011, 2015).

The genesis of TBCT was marked by the development of the Sentence Reversion-Based Thought Record (SRBTR) (de Oliveira, 2007), an adaptation of the traditional 7-column thought record designed to counter "yes, but…" types of dysfunctional thoughts (Greenberger & Padesky, 1995). These are common

I. R. de Oliveira (✉)
Federal University of Bahia, Salvador, Bahia, Brazil

A. C. Ornelas (ed.), *Transdiagnostic Approaches in Cognitive Behavioral Therapy*, https://doi.org/10.1007/978-3-031-63494-9_7

cognitive distortions where individuals negate positive feedback, reinforcing their negative beliefs. The SRBTR integrates multiple cognitive therapy techniques to help patients identify, challenge, and modify dysfunctional CBs, employing methods such as the downward arrow technique (Burns, 1980), sentence reversal (Freeman & DeWolf, 1992), and the upward arrow technique (Leahy, 2003). This comprehensive tool aims to directly confront and replace deeply entrenched negative beliefs with more adaptive, positive ones.

The transition from SRBTR to TBCT involved the introduction of a new thought record, the Trial-Based Thought Record (TBTR or Trial I), which incorporated a judicial metaphor to further aid in modifying negative CBs (Freeman & DeWolf, 1992; Leahy, 2003). This innovation showed a significant reduction in the credibility of negative CBs and the emotional distress associated with them (de Oliveira, 2008). Over time, with the incorporation of new techniques, TBCT evolved into a comprehensive therapeutic intervention, offering a unique approach to cognitive restructuring. Today, TBCT is recognized for its distinct pathway in helping patients overcome the challenges posed by dysfunctional CBs (Hemanny et al., 2023).

Similar and Distinctive Features of TBCT

TBCT aligns with conventional CBT by emphasizing a cognitive framework and fostering a collaborative therapeutic environment. It involves personalized case conceptualization, setting therapeutic goals, and integrating core CBT elements such as feedback, summaries, homework assignments, psychoeducation, and cognitive restructuring. However, TBCT distinguishes itself by introducing a unique case conceptualization diagram and a structured set of techniques across three levels and three phases of intervention. This structured approach facilitates the effective modification of ATs and the refinement of behavioral experiments to adjust intermediate beliefs, expressed as underlying assumptions (UAs). Importantly, TBCT also focuses on the transformation of CBs related to self-perception and beliefs about others. This marks a significant distinction relative to traditional CBT approaches, highlighting TBCT's unique contribution to the field of cognitive therapy (de Oliveira, 2016).

Intervention Framework

TBCT is structured to span 12–14 weekly sessions, with the flexibility to adapt to the unique needs and complexities of each case. This adaptability allows for the extension of specific techniques across more sessions if needed to enhance efficacy (de Oliveira, 2015). TBCT begins by introducing patients to the cognitive model via a conceptualization diagram. This diagram illustrates the impact of cognition on daily life and delineates three levels of information processing: Automatic thoughts (ATs) at the surface, underlying assumptions (UAs) or conditional beliefs at the intermediate level, and CBs at the deepest level. The therapeutic process in TBCT is methodically designed to address these levels, with a particular emphasis on CBs, to promote cognitive flexibility. This is supported by tools that track problems and goals throughout therapy, enhancing the therapy's efficacy and personal relevance (de Oliveira & Clyman, 2023).

Color-Coded Problem Hierarchy and Color-Coded Goals/ Aspirations Hierarchy

Within TBCT, the color-coded problems hierarchy (CCPH) and color-coded goals/ aspirations hierarchy (CCGH) function as dynamic, visual aids to streamline the therapeutic process, mapping out a patient's problems and goals in a structured and comprehensible manner (de Oliveira & Clyman, 2023).

The CCPH employs a gradient color scale, with light blue representing minor issues and red indicating severe distress. This visual scale enables therapists and patients to prioritize issues based on severity and monitor changes over time, thereby facilitating the identification of distress patterns and adjustments in therapeutic strategies.

Conversely, the CCGH uses a similar color-coding scheme but focuses on the patient's goals and aspirations. It acts as a vivid, motivational map of progress toward these aims. By visually charting the journey from lesser to greater realization of aspirations, the CCGH motivates patients to acknowledge and celebrate their progress, fostering a sense of achievement and motivation. Together, these tools not only enhance the collaborative nature of TBCT by actively involving patients in their therapy but also bridge common communication gaps, rendering abstract concepts of progress and change concrete and quantifiable.

TBCT Conceptualization Diagram

The TBCT Conceptualization Diagram is a core component of TBCT, providing a structured, step-by-step approach that divides the therapy into three levels and three phases (de Oliveira, 2012a, b). This conceptual framework is designed to flexibly accommodate the individual needs and characteristics of the patient.

Case conceptualization, a critical aspect of CBT, utilizes cognitive-behavioral theory to infer causes and maintaining factors of a patient's problems to inform interventions (Kuyken et al., 2005). The TBCT Conceptualization Diagram aims to make the cognitive model more accessible to patients and manageable for therapists, enhancing patient adherence and facilitating the therapeutic alliance.

The diagram (Fig. 7.1) illustrates the interaction between three levels of information processing within TBCT: Automatic thoughts (ATs), first level of information processing; underlying assumptions (Uas), second level of information processing; and core beliefs (CBs), third level of information processing (de Oliveira, 2012a).

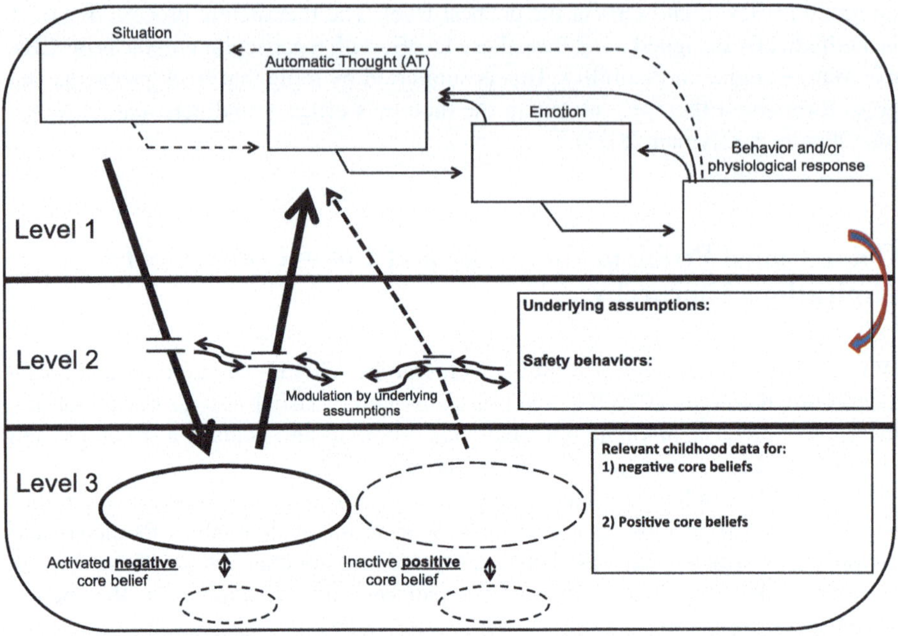

Fig. 7.1 TBCT conceptualization diagram (Phase 1, levels 1–3)

The TBCT conceptualization diagram illustrates how situation-specific behaviors, which elicit less anxiety and provide immediate relief, can evolve into safety-seeking behaviors. This transformation is represented by an arrow extending from the behavior and physiological response box at the first level to the second level. It signifies the transition from situational perceptions (ATs) to progressively becoming UAs. These UAs both sustain and are sustained by coping strategies and safety-seeking behaviors, highlighting the dynamic interplay between cognitive processes and behavioral responses (de Oliveira, 2015).

The ultimate goal of TBCT is to balance positive and negative beliefs, fostering a more adaptive engagement with functional positive CBs. The TBCT Conceptualization Diagram acts as a visual tool, aiding patients in recognizing the interplay between their thoughts, emotions, and behaviors. It guides the therapeutic process in identifying and modifying dysfunctional cognitions across all three levels, emphasizing the development and reinforcement of positive, functional CBs.

Interventions Targeting the First Level of Information Processing

At the first level of cognitive processing, ATs trigger emotional responses, leading to potentially unwanted actions, such as the fear reaction to public speaking at work. These ATs constitute the foundational layer of cognitive processing, showcasing the cyclical interaction between a situation, the resulting thought, and the consequent emotion. This cycle highlights the inherent challenge in reassessing and altering one's perceptions. Early in the therapeutic process, TBCT, paralleling standard CBT, prioritizes the identification and modification of these ATs. Since ATs are manifestations of deeper CBs, addressing them provides a direct route to correcting cognitive distortions. This approach is deemed more straightforward than directly confronting the more intricate and entrenched biases that influence an individual's perception of themselves and their interaction with the world (de Oliveira, 2012a). The subsequent sections will introduce TBCT techniques aimed at transforming these ATs.

Cognitive Distortions Questionnaire (CD-Quest)

The CD-Quest serves as an important instrument within CBT and TBCT, facilitating patient recognition of cognitive errors (de Oliveira et al., 2015; Morrison et al., 2015). This tool enables practitioners to perform a quantitative evaluation and monitor the progression of cognitive errors in patients over time. Empirical investigations have validated the CD-Quest's psychometric robustness, evidencing its internal reliability and concurrent validity across diverse studies. Its application has been effectively extended to academic environments across various countries, including Brazil (de Oliveira et al., 2015), the United States (Morrison et al., 2015; Kaplan et al., 2017), Australia (Kostoglou & Pidgeon, 2016), Turkey (Batmaz et al., 2015), and China (Qian et al., 2020).

Moreover, clinical populations in the United States (Kaplan et al., 2017) and Turkey (Batmaz et al., 2015) have been subject to studies employing the CD-Quest, further corroborating its psychometric integrity. In a pursuit of adaptability and inclusivity, recent developments have introduced abbreviated forms of the CD-Quest (Morrison et al., 2022) alongside an adaptation for adolescent populations (de Souza et al., 2023).

Intrapersonal Thought Record (Intra-TR)

The Intra-TR, an innovative tool within the TBCT framework, aids in modifying ATs (de Oliveira, 2015). It stands out by integrating first-level elements of the TBCT conceptualization diagram, offering consistency and familiarity for patients. The tool guides patients through targeted questions to clarify alternative thoughts, facilitating precise identification and modification of dysfunctional ATs. Additionally, it promotes memorization of these questions, thereby simplifying usage. This memorization helps patients internalize the process, enabling easier application of the techniques in daily scenarios.

The Intra-TR consists of 14 questions that lead the patient through a systematic process of identifying and challenging negative ATs (see Fig. 7.2). This process

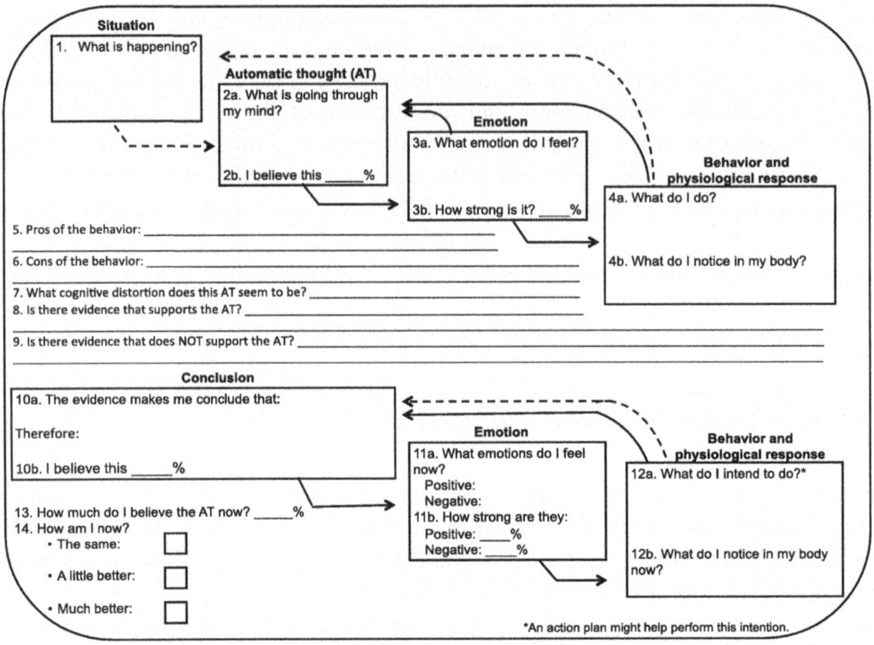

Fig. 7.2 TBCT intrapersonal thought record (Intra-TR)

includes recognizing the situation, identifying the automatic thoughts and emotions associated with it, evaluating the evidence for and against these thoughts, and then formulating a more balanced perspective. The tool also prompts patients to consider the behaviors and physical sensations that accompany their thoughts and feelings, as well as to identify the cognitive distortions at play.

In summary, the goal of using the Intra-TR is to facilitate a deeper understanding of the interplay between thoughts, emotions, and behaviors, and to foster more adaptive responses to challenging situations. By working through the Intra-TR with a therapist, and then by themselves, patients can develop a more nuanced understanding of their cognitive processes and learn to counteract negative patterns with more constructive and realistic thoughts and behaviors.

Interpersonal Thought Record (Inter-TR)

The Inter-TR is a strategic tool within TBCT designed to address interpersonal issues, enhancing patients' understanding of how their behaviors influence others and vice versa. This tool is instrumental in helping patients gain control over their behaviors, making it particularly beneficial in scenarios such as couples' therapy and for individuals suffering from social anxiety disorder. The Inter-TR facilitates the exploration of the dynamic interplay between one's actions and the reactions of others, thus providing a structured method for patients to reflect on and modify their interpersonal interactions (de Oliveira, 2016).

The process involves patients documenting specific interpersonal situations, identifying ATs that arise in these contexts, and evaluating the emotions, physical sensations, and behaviors that result from these thoughts. By examining the possible thoughts and feelings of others involved in the interaction, and by organizing an action plan, patients can develop a more nuanced understanding of the situation. This reflective practice encourages patients to consider alternative perspectives and behavior experiments, aiming to break cycles of negative interactions and improve communication and relationship dynamics.

In summary, the Inter-TR serves as a practical approach for patients to exercise more control over their interpersonal behaviors, contributing to more effective and fulfilling relationships (see Fig. 7.3). Through this guided introspection, patients can learn to navigate interpersonal conflicts more constructively, fostering a greater sense of empathy and understanding in their interactions with others.

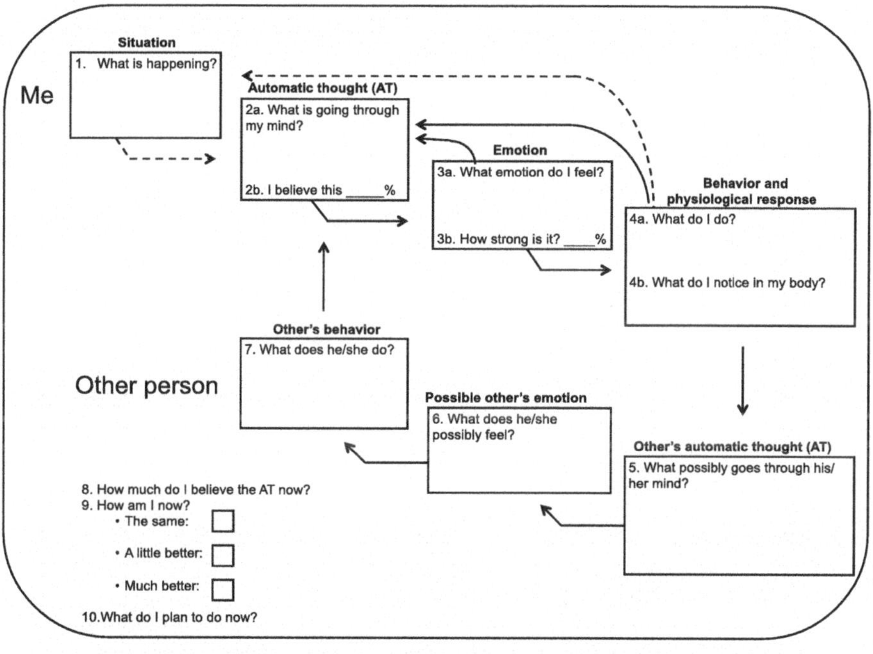

Fig. 7.3 TBCT interpersonal thought record (Inter-TR)

Participation Grid (PG)

The PG represents a nuanced approach within TBCT aimed at addressing and resolving feelings of guilt and shame (de Oliveira, 2016). This method innovatively builds upon and advances beyond traditional techniques, such as the responsibility pie used in CBT, by offering a structured framework for patients to gradually expose themselves to and reassess their involvement in guilt-inducing events. Unlike its predecessors, the PG introduces a methodical way for individuals to evaluate their perceived contribution towards an adverse situation, often leading to the realization that their actual participation is significantly less than initially believed. This reassessment process not only diminishes feelings of guilt and shame but also promotes a transformative understanding of personal responsibility that is more in line with the individual's values and commitments.

Through the PG, patients are guided to methodically list all entities, including themselves, that may have played a role in the event, subsequently assigning a perceived percentage of contribution to each (see Fig. 7.4). This exercise frequently culminates in a profound reevaluation of self-blame, as individuals discover their part to be less or sometimes minimal, thereby alleviating excessive guilt. Moreover,

I believe I am ______% guilty for______________________________

PARTICIPATION

Participation Assessment	1st Evaluation	2nd Evaluation	3rd Evaluation	4th Evaluation	5th Evaluation
Myself					
Total Percentage	100	100	100	100	100

I believe I am ______% guilty for______________________________

Fig. 7.4 Participation grid

this reassessment encourages a shift from a guilt-centric viewpoint to a participation-focused perspective, facilitating a path towards repairing that emphasizes proactive engagement with personal values and commitments. Thus, the PG not only serves as a therapeutic tool for mitigating unwarranted feelings of guilt and shame but also as a catalyst for fostering a deeper sense of self-compassion and resilience among patients.

Interventions Targeting the Second Level of Information Processing

In TBCT, particular emphasis is placed on the intermediate level of information processing, which concerns the identification and modification of rules, underlying assumptions, or conditional beliefs that patients hold (de Oliveira, 2012a). Therapists employ the TBCT conceptualization diagram as a crucial tool in this process. This approach educates patients to understand how certain habitual behaviors, referred to as safety-seeking behaviors, contribute to the perpetuation of specific perceptions through confirmatory bias. These perceptions gradually solidify into rigid rules or underlying assumptions (de Oliveira, 2015). By changing such behaviors with behavioral experiments, TBCT aims to interrupt these reinforcing cycles, promoting cognitive restructuring and leading to healthier thought patterns and behaviors (De Oliveira, 2012a).

Thus, behavioral experiments play a pivotal role in TBCT by being especially efficacious for identifying and changing the rules and assumptions that underlie cognitive processes at the intermediate level (Bennett-Levy et al., 2010). These experiments serve as a practical method for patients to directly test the validity of their conditional beliefs and assumptions against real-world experiences. By engaging in behavioral experiments, patients can observe firsthand the discrepancies between their expectations and actual outcomes, which is instrumental for cognitive restructuring at this level (Greenberger & Padesky, 1995). Consequently, these experiments are not only fundamental for challenging and modifying intermediate-level cognitive structures but are also crucial for altering dysfunctional cognitions across the other levels of information processing. This hands-on approach facilitates a profound and lasting change in the way patients perceive and interact with their environment, leading to more adaptive and healthy cognitive patterns.

Despite the logical underpinnings of these interventions being clear to the patient, clinicians often find it necessary to introduce additional strategies to address any ambivalence the patient may experience towards experiments involving exposure to varying degrees (Rouf et al., 2010). In TBCT, we add the color-coded symptom hierarchy (CCSH) and the consensual role-play (CRP).

Color-Coded Symptom Hierarchy

The CCSH (de Oliveira, 2016) is a novel approach to enhance engagement in behavioral experiments. It allows patients to visually map out and confront their symptoms based on the level of discomfort or distress they cause. By categorizing symptoms into color-coded levels—green for manageable discomfort, yellow for significant distress necessitating therapist support, and red for overwhelming distressing symptoms not to be challenged, at least temporarily—patients can strategically plan their exposures. This method not only aids in the gradual confrontation of fears but also in the reevaluation of perceived threats, leading to a noticeable decrease in symptom intensity over time, including those initially deemed most daunting (red symptoms).

Consensual Role-Play (CRP)

The CRP stands out as a therapeutic intervention for tackling ambivalence, particularly in scenarios where patients grapple with conflicting internal narratives due to entrenched safety behaviors and the underlying assumptions that maintain them. This method meticulously dissects the dichotomy between reason and emotion, paving the way for a synthesized, consensus-driven self-view (Greenberger & Padesky, 1995). The seven-step CRP process is meticulously designed to foster introspection and exploration, rather than hastening towards a decision. After carefully evaluating the advantages and disadvantages of a feared or desired action, assigning relative importance to each argument, and engaging in a dialogue between contrasting viewpoints by means of the "empty chair" approach, CRP enables individuals to navigate their internal conflicts towards a "consensual" resolution (de Oliveira, 2015). The technique culminates in an action plan tailored to the patient's readiness to confront or delay the action, thereby equipping them with a strategic approach to decision-making (see Fig. 7.5). This process not only demystifies the decision-making labyrinth but also empowers patients to approach their dilemmas with a renewed sense of clarity and purpose.

The "empty chair" approach is a crucial element of CRP, facilitating dialogue between the patient's conflicting rational and emotional perspectives. This technique is instrumental in fostering internal consensus, allowing patients to directly externalize and confront their ambivalence. Through this interactive process, patients are guided towards gaining insights and achieving a balanced understanding, which supports a unified self-perception and informed decision-making (de Oliveira, 2012a).

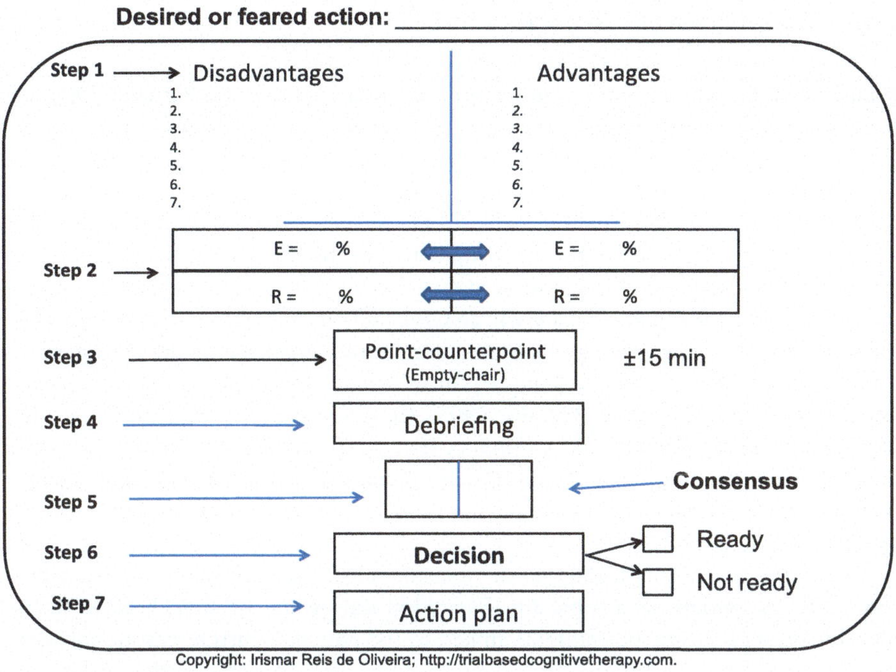

Fig. 7.5 Consensual role-play (CRP)

Interventions Targeting the Third Level of Information Processing

In CBT, interventions targeting the third level of information processing focus on the modification of dysfunctional negative CBs (Wenzel, 2012). CBs are deeply held convictions that shape our interpretation of ourselves, others, and the world (Beck, 1976). CBs often emerge from our early life experiences and influence our thoughts, emotions, and behaviors in profound and continuous ways. By addressing them, therapists aim to facilitate lasting change in patients' psychological patterns, promoting healthier coping mechanisms and a more adaptive behavior (Beck, 2011). In TBCT, we use the Negative Core Beliefs Inventory (NCBI), as developed by Osmo et al. (2018), to identify, assess and keep track of dysfunctional negative CBs about oneself and others. Below, we outline strategies and techniques specifically aimed at modifying dysfunctional negative CBs, a crucial aspect of TBCT.

Trial-Based Thought Record (Trial I)

Trial I or TBTR is the primary intervention strategy of TBCT (de Oliveira, 2012b). It facilitates the identification of self-directed criticisms as expressions of the activation of negative CBs rather than incontrovertible realities. This process allows the formulation of a reasonable defense strategy, drawing a contrast to the fate of Joseph K. in the allegorical narrative by Kafka in his novel carrying the same name, The Trial (Kafka, 1925/1998). Trial I is distinguished from other CB interventions for its methodical and sequential integration of a variety of techniques that have been previously validated for their efficacy within CBT and other therapeutic modalities (de Oliveira, 2015). These techniques include the empty chair technique (Carstenson, 1955), the downward arrow technique (Burns, 1980), the examination of evidence (Beck, 2011; Greenberger & Padesky, 1995), the defense attorney metaphor (Leahy, 2003; Freeman & DeWolf, 1992), sentence reversal (Freeman & DeWolf, 1992), the upward arrow technique (Leahy, 2003; de Oliveira, 2012b), the development of a positive schema (Leahy, 2003), the positive data log (Beck, 2011), and letter writing (Pennebaker & Beall, 1986).

The initial use of this technique involves the clinician addressing the issue presented by the patient as a topic for discussion during the session. Following the identification of automatic thoughts linked to the patient's current emotional state, the clinician employs the downward arrow technique to uncover the underlying negative CB, referred to here as "self-accusation." This step includes determining the patient's level of conviction in this self-view and the strength of the related emotional response (Table 7.1, Column 1).

Table 7.1 TBCT form (Trial I)

Please, briefly describe the situation: ……………………………………………………………………

1. **Inquiry/Establishing the accusation (core belief).** What was going through your mind before you started to feel this way? Ask yourself what these thoughts meant about yourself, supposing they were true. The answer "*If these thoughts were true, it means I am a …*" is the uncovered **self-accusation** (core belief).	2. **Prosecutor's plea.** Please, state all the evidence you have that **supports** the accusation/core belief that you have circled in column 1.	3. **Defense attorney's plea:** Please, state all the evidence you have that **does not support** the accusation/core belief that you have circled in column 1.	4. **Prosecutor's rebuttal to the defendant's plea.** Please, state the thoughts that question, discount, or disqualify each piece of positive evidence in column 3, usually expressed as "yes, but…" thoughts.	5. **Defense attorney's rejoinder to the prosecutor's plea.** Please, after reading each thought of column 4, add the conjunction BUT, and then provide the meaning about you. **Note**: columns 5 and 6 are filled in at the same time.	6. **Conclusion about the meaning.** Please, state your conclusion after the conjunction **therefore**.	7. **Juror's verdict.** Please, report cognitive distortions made by the prosecutor and the defense attorney and give the verdict.
Downward arrow technique: *If the thoughts above were true, what would they mean about you?* ↓ *I am ………*	*1)* *2)* *3)* *4)* *5)* *6)*	*1)* *2)* *3)* *4)* *5)* *6)*	**But:** *1)* *2)* *3)* *4)* *5)* *6)*	**Meaning:** *1)* *2)* *3)* *4)* *5)* *6)*	**Therefore:** *1)* *2)* *3)* *4)* *5)* *6)*	**Cognitive distortions:** **Prosecutor 1**: 1 - 2 - 3 - 4 - 5 - 6 - **Defense 1**: 1 - 2 - 3 - 4 - 5 - 6 - **Prosecutor 2**: 1 - 2 - 3 - 4 - 5 - 6 - **Defense 2**: 1 - 2 - 3 - 4 - 5 - 6 - **Verdict:**
Now, how much (%) do you believe you are …………? **Initial: Final:** What **emotion** does this belief make you feel? ………… How strong (%) is it? **Initial: Final:**	Now, how much (%) do you believe you are ………? ………% How strong (%) is your ……………now? ………%	Now, how much (%) do you believe you are ………? ………% How strong (%) is your ……………now? ………%	Now, how much (%) do you believe you are ………? ………% How strong (%) is your ……………now? ………%		Now, how much (%) do you believe you are ………? ………% How strong (%) is your ……………now? ………%	Now, how much (%) do you believe you are ………? ………% How strong (%) is your ……………now? ………%

The subsequent columns are delineated by the roles of the prosecutor and the defense attorney. These roles alternately argue in support of and against the negative CB that constitutes the basis of the patient's self-accusation (Column 2). The prosecutor's arguments often introduce new ATs, mostly distorted, that serve to perpetuate the patient's negative self-perception. It is also typical for patients to express skepticism towards the arguments presented by the defense (Column 3). Nonetheless, the effectiveness of a defense attorney is not contingent upon their personal belief in the client's innocence but rather on their capability to rigorously gather evidence that brings reasonable doubt that leads to the client verdict of not guilty.

The fourth column is specifically allocated for the prosecutor's counterarguments, which aim to invalidate, disqualify or diminish the defense's claims using the conjunction "but." This often results in the emergence of more ATs–the same the patients use in their everyday life– that sustain the negative CB (Column 4).

In a similar vein, the defense's response registered in Columns 5 and 6, leverages the same logic, prompting the patient to reverse the sequence of arguments presented in the third and fourth columns, again connected by the conjunction "but." This reversal of the phrase allows the patient to view the scenario from a more optimistic and accurate standpoint, an understanding that is deepened by exploring its significance to the patient.

Mirroring the judicial process, the subsequent phase involves the jury's verdict (Column 7), serving as the evaluative component of the therapy. Here, the patient, acting as a juror, is tasked with assessing the effectiveness of both the prosecution and defense. This assessment involves considering the arguments' coherence and substance, their grounding in factual evidence, the presence or absence of intention behind actions, and, most importantly, the utilization of cognitive distortions in reaching a verdict on the accusation.

It is important to note that the intensity of the belief and the related emotion are reassessed and documented following each character's presentation (Columns 1 through 7), thereby reinforcing the TBCT framework.

Upon the proclamation of the verdict, the therapist and the patient transition from the "judicial setting" back to the "therapeutic setting." At this point, the therapist utilizes the upward arrow technique (de Oliveira, 2007) to foster the activation of the patient's functional positive belief system. In scenarios where the judgment typically favors the defendant—the patient—they are prompted with the question, "Assuming your defense attorney is correct and the jury has made a fair decision, what does this imply about you?" This question initiates the next phase, which includes preparation for a potential appeal by the prosecution, a step taken even in the uncommon event of the defendant's guilt being affirmed.

The positive data log functions as making the defense attorney an ally in this context. The patient is instructed to systematically collect evidence supporting the newly formed positive belief over the following week, effectively countering the prosecution's charges (the patient's daily life distorted by active negative CBs). This regimen entails a daily evaluation of the patient's confidence in the positive affirmation, quantified in percentages, starting within the therapy session itself as part of the "preparation for the appeal" exercise. Additionally, during the same session, after assessing the patient's belief in the positive statement, a reevaluation of the negative belief is performed, with the findings recorded at the bottom of the first column on the Trial I form.

Trial-Based Metacognitive Awareness (Trial II)

In more severe instances, characterized by the heightened susceptibility of the patient's negative CBs to activation, it may transpire that new instances of self-accusation emerge even following multiple successes by the defense attorney. Under such circumstances, employing Trial II can prove to be particularly beneficial. This stage affords the patient the unique chance to levy accusations against the prosecutor, charging them with incompetence, abuse, or harassment, in light of the considerable harm and losses inflicted across various aspects of the patient's life. By this phase, the patient will have developed the ability to gain perspective on and reflect upon their thoughts (metacognition), rendering the prosecutor's assertions significantly less persuasive (de Oliveira, 2012b, 2015). This shift marks a critical evolution in the therapeutic process, where the patient begins to assert control over previously uncontested negative narratives. At this juncture, the patient becomes the judge of his or her own life, adjudicating over the validity and influence of negative CBs.

Sailboat Metaphor

The "Sailboat Metaphor" is employed in TBCT to bolster resilience and empower patients to navigate through challenging situations. This metaphor stands out as a unique practical element during relaxation exercises, aimed at clarifying and strengthening the patient's understanding of metacognition. It likens thoughts to the wind, emotions to the waves, and behavior to steering the rudder. The act of adjusting the sail, either by hoisting or lowering it, symbolizes metacognitive awareness. This implies that in tranquil conditions, one may let thoughts pass without engagement (hoisting the sail), whereas in tumultuous times, it's possible to assess thoughts critically and choose not to act on them (lowering the sail). Employing this metaphor highlights the impermanent nature of thoughts and emotions, cultivating a sense of mastery and perspective over one's mental activities (de Oliveira, 2015).

Applications of TBCT and Empirical Data

In the foundational study conducted by de Oliveira in 2008, 30 participants demonstrated significant reductions in the intensity of beliefs and emotional distress. Further research with a larger sample (n = 166) reinforced these results, establishing the TBTR as an effective tool within TBCT for diminishing negative CBs and reducing self-criticism, thereby highlighting its value in altering dysfunctional beliefs and emotions (de Oliveira et al., 2012a).

In a subsequent randomized trial, de Oliveira et al. (2012b) assessed the TBTR's efficacy against conventional CBT in treating Social Anxiety Disorder (SAD), finding the TBTR more effective in decreasing fear of negative evaluation among SAD patients. Further analysis by Powell et al. (2013) on the same dataset revealed significant improvements in Quality of Life (QoL) indicators, including general health, vitality, and mental health in SAD patients. These findings emphasize the TBTR's superiority not only in addressing CBs but also in enhancing QoL, indicating its wider applicability in managing emotional disorders.

Caetano et al. (2018) explored the efficacy of TBCT for treating Generalized Social Anxiety Disorder (SAD) with comorbid depression in a randomized clinical trial involving 39 adults, comparing TBCT to a waitlist control group. Participants in the TBCT group exhibited significant reductions in social anxiety, social avoidance, and depression, underscoring TBCT's effectiveness, especially for patients with comorbid conditions. This study bolstered TBCT as a promising approach for SAD, emphasizing its capability to address both social anxiety and depressive symptoms efficiently.

Hemanny et al. (2020) examined the efficacy of TBCT, Behavioral Activation (BA), and Treatment as Usual (TAU) for Major Depressive Disorder (MDD) in a clinical trial. The study revealed that TBCT and BA, when combined with antidepressants, were more effective than TAU (antidepressants alone) in diminishing depressive symptoms and disability. This finding suggests that integrating TBCT or BA with standard antidepressant treatment could enhance clinical outcomes for MDD. A subsequent analysis (Hemanny et al., 2021) of the same dataset indicated that adding BA and TBCT to antidepressant treatment might reduce suicidal ideation. This research, notable for its focus on BA and being the first to assess the impact of TBCT on suicidal ideation, highlighted the clinical significance of these therapies in managing suicidality among MDD patients, suggesting these psychotherapeutic interventions as valuable adjuncts to pharmacotherapy in the treatment of depression.

Duran et al. (2021) evaluated the efficacy of TBCT against Prolonged Exposure (PE) therapy in treating Post-Traumatic Stress Disorder (PTSD). Both therapies demonstrated significant reductions in PTSD symptoms, yet no notable differences were observed between the two. However, TBCT was associated with greater improvements in depressive symptoms and exhibited a lower dropout rate than PE, indicating TBCT's potential as a viable alternative to PE for PTSD, particularly for its benefits in comorbid depression and improving patient retention.

Rodrigues et al. (2023) investigated TBCT's efficacy compared to Exposure and Response Prevention (ERP) in treating obsessive-compulsive disorder (OCD). Both treatments significantly reduced OCD symptom severity, with no significant differences detected between them. This study highlighted TBCT's promise as an effective treatment for OCD, with therapeutic gains sustained at a 12-month follow-up.

Lastly, a systematic review and meta-analysis by Hemanny et al. (2023), evaluating TBCT's efficacy and dropout rates for treating depressive and anxious symptoms against other psychotherapies, included ten randomized clinical trials (RCTs) with 1245 participants. The results indicated that TBCT is comparably effective to other leading psychotherapies for symptom reduction, exhibiting similar dropout rates. This analysis accentuated TBCT's adaptability and applicability across various mental health conditions and settings, proposing it as a promising alternative within the psychotherapeutic intervention spectrum. However, the authors called for further rigorous and geographically diverse research to validate these findings.

Future Perspectives on TBCT

As TBCT continues to establish itself as a transdiagnostic and effective therapeutic approach, the horizon for its application and research holds promising potential. Accumulated empirical evidence underscores TBCT's efficacy across a spectrum of emotional disorders, including anxiety, depression, PTSD, and OCD, highlighting its adaptability and significant impact on patients' lives. Innovations in TBCT are anticipated to enhance its integration with technological advances, such as digital mental health platforms, and to incorporate mindfulness practices. This integrated focus aims to increase accessibility and engagement, offering a more holistic approach to treatment. The inclusion of mindfulness practices in particular promises to enrich TBCT's therapeutic toolkit, facilitating a deeper engagement with the present moment and enhancing emotional regulation across diverse patient populations.

The challenge and opportunity moving forward involve expanding the empirical base through more rigorous, geographically diverse research to solidify TBCT's standing and uncover its full potential. Further exploration into the nuances of its application across different cultures and populations will enrich TBCT's transdiagnostic utility and efficacy, ensuring that it remains a relevant and powerful tool in the mental health professional's arsenal.

As mental health professionals continue to refine and adapt TBCT, it stands well-positioned to broaden its therapeutic reach and deepen our understanding of cognitive therapy's capacity for transformation. The future holds the potential for a landscape where nuanced, personalized therapy becomes increasingly accessible and effective, offering the promise of enhanced outcomes for individuals facing a wide range of emotional disorders.

References

Batmaz, S., Kocbiyik, S., & Yuncu, O. A. (2015). Turkish version of the Cognitive Distortions Questionnaire: Psychometric properties. *Depression Research and Treatment, 2015*, 1–8.

Beck, A. T. (1976). *Cognitive therapy and the emotional disorders*. International University Press.

Beck, J. S. (2011). *Cognitive behavior therapy: Basics and beyond* (2nd ed.). Guilford Press.

Bennett-Levy, J., Westbrook, D., Fennell, M., Cooper, M., Rouf, K., & Hackmann, A. (2010). Behavioural experiments: Historical and conceptual underpinnings. In J. Bennett-Levy, G. Butler, M. Fennell, A. Hackmann, M. Mueller, & D. Westbrook (Eds.), *Oxford guide to behavioural experiments in cognitive therapy*. Oxford University Press.

Burns, D. D. (1980). *Feeling good: The new mood therapy*. Harper Collins Publishers.

Caetano, K. A. S., Depreeuw, B., Papenfuss, I., Curtiss, J., Langwerden, R. J., Hofmann, S. G., & Neufeld, C. B. (2018). Trial-Based Cognitive Therapy: Efficacy of a new CBT approach for treating social anxiety disorder with comorbid depression. *International Journal of Cognitive Therapy, 11*(3), 325–342. https://doi.org/10.1007/s41811-018-0028-7

Carstenson, B. (1955). The auxiliary chair technique—A case study. *Group Psychotherapy, 8*, 50–56.

de Oliveira, I. R. (2007). Sentence reversion-based thought record (SRBTR): A new strategy to deal with 'yes, but...' dysfunctional thoughts in cognitive therapy. *European Review of Applied Psychology, 57*, 17–22.

de Oliveira, I. R. (2008). Trial-based thought record (TBTR): Preliminary data on a strategy to deal with core beliefs by combining sentence reversion and the use of an analogy to a trial. *Revista Brasileira de Psiquiatria, 30*(1), 12–18.

de Oliveira, I. R. (2011). Kafka's trial dilemma: Proposal of a practical solution to Joseph K's unknown accusation. *Medical Hypotheses, 77*(1), 5–6.

de Oliveira, I. R. (2012a). Assessing and restructuring dysfunctional cognitions. In I. R. de Oliveira (Ed.), *Standard and innovative strategies in cognitive behavior therapy*. InTech. Available from: http://www.intechopen.com/books/standard-and-innovative-strategies-in-cognitive-behavior-therapy

de Oliveira, I. R. (2012b). Use of the Trial-Based Thought Record to change negative core beliefs. In I. R. de Oliveira (Ed.), *Standard and innovative strategies in cognitive behavior therapy*. InTech. Available from: http://www.intechopen.com/books/standard-and-innovative-strategies-in-cognitive-behavior-therapy

de Oliveira, I. R. (2015). *Trial-based cognitive therapy: A manual for clinicians* (Clinical topics in psychology and psychiatry). Routledge.

de Oliveira, I. R. (2016). *Trial-based cognitive therapy: Distinctive features*. Routledge.

de Oliveira, I. R., & Clyman, N. (2023). Color-coded problems hierarchy (CCPH) and color-coded goals/aspirations hierarchy (CCGH): Quantitative approaches to tracking progress in cognitive behavior therapy. *Advances in CBT, Winter Issue*, 13–17.

de Oliveira, I. R., Hemanny, C., Powell, V. B., Bonfim, T. D., Duran, E. P., Novais, N. S. S. M., Velasquez, M., Di Sarno, E., Alves, G. L., Cesnik, J. A., & the Brazilian TBTR Study Group. (2012a). Trial-based psychotherapy and the efficacy of trial-based thought record in changing unhelpful core beliefs and reducing self-criticism. *CNS Spectrums, 17*(1), 16–23. https://doi.org/10.1017/S1092852912000399

de Oliveira, I. R., Powell, V. B., Wenzel, A., Caldas, M., Seixas, C., Almeida, C., Bonfim, T. D., Grangeon, M. C., Castro, M., Galvão, A., Moraes, R. O., & Sudak, D. M. (2012b). Efficacy of the trial-based thought record, a new cognitive therapy strategy designed to change core beliefs in social phobia. *Journal of Clinical Pharmacy and Therapeutics, 37*, 328–334. https://doi.org/10.1111/j.1365-2710.2011.01300.x

de Oliveira, I. R., Seixas, C., Osório, F. L., Crippa, J. A. S., Abreu, J. N., Menezes, I. G., et al. (2015). Evaluation of the psychometric properties of the cognitive distortions questionnaire (CD-Quest) in a sample of undergraduate students. *Innovations in Clinical Neuroscience, 12*(7–8), 20–27.

de Souza, C. L. S. G., Pires, P. P., Couto, I. S. L., de Vasconcelos, N. S. S. M., Menezes, I. G., & de Oliveira, I. R. (2023). Development and psychometric properties of the Cognitive Distortions Questionnaire for Adolescents (CD-Quest-T). *Trends in Psychiatry and Psychotherapy, 45*, e20210214. https://doi.org/10.47626/2237-6089-2021-0214

Duran, É. P., Corchs, F., Vianna, A., Araújo, Á. C., Del Real, N., Silva, C., Ferreira, A. P., De Vitto Francez, P., Godói, C., Silveira, H., Matsumoto, L., Gebara, C. M., de Barros Neto, T. P., Chilvarquer, R., de Siqueira, L. L., Bernik, M., & Neto, F. L. (2021). A randomized clinical trial to assess the efficacy of trial-based cognitive therapy compared to prolonged exposure for post-traumatic stress disorder: Preliminary findings. *CNS Spectrums, 26*(4), 427–434. https://doi.org/10.1017/S1092852920001455

Freeman, A., & DeWolf, R. (1992). *The 10 dumbest mistakes smart people make and how to avoid them*. HyperPerennial.

Greenberger, D., & Padesky, C. A. (1995). *Mind over mood: Change how you feel by changing the way you think*. Guilford Press.

Hemanny, C., Carvalho, C., Maia, N., Reis, D., Botelho, A. C., Bonavides, D., Seixas, C., & de Oliveira, I. R. (2020). Efficacy of trial-based cognitive therapy, behavioral activation, and treatment as usual in the treatment of major depressive disorder: Preliminary findings from a randomized clinical trial. *CNS Spectrums, 25*(4), 535–544. https://doi.org/10.1017/S1092852919001457

Hemanny, C., de Sena Pondé, E., & de Oliveira, I. R. (2021). Behavioural activation and trial-based cognitive therapy may be beneficial to reduce suicidal ideation in major depressive disorder: A post hoc study from a clinical trial. *Journal of Clinical Pharmacy and Therapeutics, 46*(2), 516–523. https://doi.org/10.1111/jcpt.13335

Hemanny, C., dos Santos, C. O., Moris, F. T. L., & Melnik, T. (2023). Trial-Based Cognitive Therapy for depressive and anxious symptoms: A systematic review and meta-analysis of efficacy and dropout rates. *Journal of Mood and Anxiety Disorders, 1*, 100005.

Kafka, F. (1925/1998). *The trial*. Schocken Books.

Kaplan, S. C., Morrison, A. S., Goldin, P. R., Olino, T. M., Heimberg, R. G., & Gross, J. J. (2017). The Cognitive Distortions Questionnaire (CD-Quest): Validation in a sample of adults with social anxiety disorder. *Cognitive Therapy and Research, 41*, 576–587.

Kostoglou, S. L., & Pidgeon, A. M. (2016). The cognitive distortions questionnaire: Psychometric validation for an Australian population. *Australian Journal of Psychology, 68*(2), 123–129.

Kuyken, W., Fothergill, C. D., Musa, M., & Chadwick, P. (2005). The reliability and quality of cognitive case formulation. *Behaviour Research and Therapy, 43*, 1187–1201.

Leahy, R. L. (2003). *Cognitive therapy techniques: A practitioner's guide*. Guilford Press.

Morrison, A. S., Potter, C. M., Carper, M. M., Kinner, D. G., Jensen, D., Bruce, L., et al. (2015). The Cognitive Distortions Questionnaire (CD-Quest): Psychometric properties and exploratory factor analysis. *International Journal of Clinical Psychology, 8*(4), 287–305.

Morrison, A. S., Ustun, B., Horenstein, A., Kaplan, S. C., de Oliveira, I. R., Batmaz, S., Gross, J. J., Sadikova, E., Hemanny, C., Pires, P. P., Goldin, P. R., Kessler, R. C., & Heimberg, R. G. (2022). Optimized short-forms of the Cognitive Distortions Questionnaire. *Journal of Anxiety Disorders, 92*, 102624.

Osmo, F., Duran, V., Wenzel, A., de Oliveira, I. R., Nepomuceno, S., Madeira, M., & Menezes, I. (2018). The Negative Core Beliefs Inventory: Development and psychometric properties. *Journal of Cognitive Psychotherapy: An International Quarterly, 32*(1), 67–84. https://doi.org/10.1891/0889-8391.32.1.67

Pennebaker, J. W., & Beall, S. K. (1986). Confronting a traumatic event: Toward an understanding of inhibition and disease. *Journal of Abnormal Psychology, 95*(3), 274–281. https://doi.org/10.1037/0021-843x.95.3.274

Powell, V. B., de Oliveira, O. H., Seixas, C., Almeida, C., Grangeon, M. C., Caldas, M., Bonfim, T. D., Castro, M., Galvão, A., Moraes, R. O., Sudak, D., & de-Oliveira, I. R. (2013). Changing core beliefs with trial-based therapy may improve quality of life in social phobia: A randomized study. *Revista Brasileira de Psiquiatria, 35*, 1–5. https://doi.org/10.1590/1516-4446-2012-0863

Qian, L., Liu, L., Chen, M., Wang, S., Cao, Z., & Zhang, N. (2020). Reliability and validity of the Chinese version of the Cognitive Distortions Questionnaire (CD-Quest) in college students. *Medical Science Monitor, 26*, e926786–1-e926786-8.

Rodrigues, E. P., Fechine, A. J. B., Oliveira, A. C., Matos, C. F. F., Passarela, C. d. M., Hemanny, C., Dias, F. d. M., Batista, J. W., Albuquerque, L. d. C. N., Soares, M. S., Neto, P. E. C., Araújo, V. P. d. C., Ayres, Z. M., & de Oliveira, I. R. (2023). Randomized trial of the efficacy of trial-based cognitive therapy for obsessive-compulsive disorder: Preliminary findings. *Trends in Psychiatry and Psychotherapy, 45*, e20210247. https://doi.org/10.47626/2237-6089-2021-0247

Rouf, K., Fennell, M., Westbrook, D., Cooper, M., & Bennett-Levy, J. (2010). Devising effective behavioural experiments. In J. Bennett-Levy, G. Butler, M. Fennell, A. Hackmann, M. Mueller, & D. Westbrook (Eds.), *Oxford guide to behavioural experiments in Cognitive Therapy*. Oxford University Press.

Wenzel, A. (2012). Modification of core beliefs in cognitive therapy. In I. R. de Oliveira (Ed.), *Standard and innovative strategies in cognitive behavior therapy*. InTech. Available from: http://www.intechopen.com/books/standard-and-innovative-strategies-in-cognitive-behavior-therapy

Chapter 8
Acceptance and Commitment Therapy (ACT)

Veruska Andrea Santos and Fernanda Coutinho

Introduction

Acceptance and Commitment Therapy (ACT) was developed by Steven Hayes in the late 1980s, but only in 1999 did Hayes, along with Kelly Wilson and Kirk Strrosahl, publish their first manual with theory and practice. The approach emerges as a contextual behavioral therapy with the aim of modifying the way the individual deals with human suffering from psychological flexibility. (Hayes et al., 1999, 2012) ACT is considered a transdiagnostic approach, as it does not seek to treat disorders or free the individual from some specific suffering. It promotes psychological flexibility from the development of the ability to experience the present moment in an open and non-judgmental way while behaviors follow the guidance of the individual's life values (Hayes et al., 2006).

At this point, the practice of mindfulness emerges as a facilitator for psychological processes and a gateway to getting behavioral experiences. In addition to mindfulness, ACT bases its interventions on acceptance and commitment to valuable actions. (Hayes, 2004) According to Hayes, experiential avoidance is the origin of emotional problems, as it not only limits behavioral responses, but directs them so that the individual does not suffer or feel pain, thus he cannot direct his behaviors towards what is valuable. He is always in the direction of reducing suffering or doing something to avoid suffering (Fletcher & Hayes, 2005), potentially becoming responsible for the development and maintenance of psychopathologies (Hayes et al., 2006).

V. A. Santos (✉)
Tijuca, RJ, Brazil

F. Coutinho
Leblon, RJ, Brazil; http://www.catc.com.br

A. C. Ornelas (ed.), *Transdiagnostic Approaches in Cognitive Behavioral Therapy*, https://doi.org/10.1007/978-3-031-63494-9_8

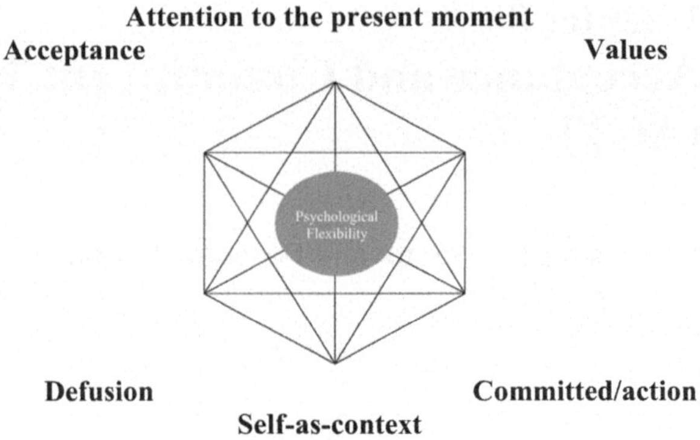

Fig. 8.1 Hexagon model of flexibility

In the opposite direction of avoidance and experiential evasion reinforced by Western society, Hayes emphasizes that psychological suffering caused by thoughts, memories, and feelings should be seen as something natural and part of the human condition. He also emphasizes that refuting experiences considered painful (experiential avoidance) is a basic and evolutionary human instinct, however it intensifies suffering (Hayes et al., 2006, 2012a).

The approach proposes to create opportunities and space for the individual to come into contact with all human experiences and change their relationship with them. (Hayes et al., 2006, 2012a) Psychological flexibility is achieved through six psychological dimensions. These skills/processes are organized into a set of interdependent competencies, illustrated in a hexagonal format, and each vertex corresponds to a specific skill. Hayes named it the Hexaflex model (Saban, 2015). The Hexaflex can organize these dimensions and direct the evaluation and intervention in ACT. The Hexaflex can be understood as a visual resource to organize, synthesize, and clarify what is contributing to the individual's suffering (Wilson et al., 2012). Intervention strategies use functional analyses, metaphors, and structured exercises in each of the psychological processes of the illustration. Figure 8.1: Illustration of the hexagon model of psychological flexibility (Hayes et al., 2012a).

It is valid to note that the six processes are equally necessary for the individual to achieve psychological flexibility. According to the authors, no process is superior and there is no defined order for them to be worked on in psychotherapy. The rule is that all are worked on, and the functional analysis of the individual context will indicate which dimension will be worked on at each moment of treatment (Hayes et al., 2012a).

Acceptance

The dimension of *acceptance* is the dimension of affect, of longing to feel, which has as its contrary and pathological response, experiential avoidance. Acceptance involves the way the individual deals with feelings. It involves the ability to tolerate discomfort and to engage in responses caused by his history, actively and consciously, without attempts to change the frequency, form, or course. To accept, for ACT, involves making room for what happens in the present moment and, for this, training in mindfulness is essential, as it makes the psychological dimension of acceptance exist in a more objective and practical way. The intention is to be open to emotions and accept human experiences in their entirety, whether they are "pleasant" or not. ACT assumes that the rational mind classifies emotions as good or bad and determines, in this way, which emotions should be avoided or controlled. Therefore, it is important to understand this classification to learn to observe in a gentle and conscious way the feeling in all its amplitude of possibilities. Understanding feeling as an attribute of humanity, and with the practice of mindfulness, it is possible to develop acceptance of emotions and feelings as part of a full life (Harris, 2011).

Hayes endorses this idea by writing "Emotions are not the problem they are just messengers and the messages they carry need to be heard, as they often show us opportunities".

In order to enrich the acceptance process, the metaphor of the unwanted guest ("Joe the Bum"), presented in the original ACT book of 1999, is an excellent resource to illustrate evasion and acceptance.

Unwanted Guest Metaphor (Adapted from Hayes et al., 1999, pp. 239–240)

Imagine that you have moved and are in a new neighborhood and a new house. Because of this, you invited all your neighbors to an "open house" reception, after all, connecting with people nearby is important to you. You even posted an invitation on the wall of a nearby supermarket that everyone frequents. The party started and all the neighbors arrived including John, a homeless man, who lives behind the market next to a dump. John is always dirty, poorly dressed, and stinking, and when you see him at your party you think: "I can't believe he's here", but the invitation pinned on the market wall said, "everyone is invited!" Only at that moment do you realize that not everyone was welcome, and John was not. But as soon as you realize all this, your party changes. You encourage him to leave, but when you get distracted, he returns. So, you stand guard at the house door to make sure he won't be able to return. Meanwhile, life is happening and moving forward, just like the party (and along with it, what was originally important to you: connecting with your neighbors) but you are missing the party and the possibility of meeting your neighbors, because you are stuck in the fight against John's presence! So, you decide to change and let him in even though you don't like his presence. You manage to greet him and receive him even though you don't want to and don't like what you're doing. But you decide to stop fighting and realize that you don't need to like him, how he dresses, or his smell. You notice that your evaluations and opinions about him are different from your willingness to invite him to your house. In this way, you finally realize that by accepting him in your house, you free yourself up to enjoy the party and connect with the neighbors, which was the initial goal of having promoted the party, bringing you closer to the life you want to live. (Adapted from Hayes et al., 1999, pp. 239–240).

To promote acceptance in clinical practice, it is necessary for the patient to not only notice what happens in the present moment, but to choose to stay in it. For this, mindfulness training can and should be used so that the patient perceives and comes into contact with internal stimuli (Araújo et al., 2021; Lucena-Santos et al., 2021).

Cognitive Defusion

The psychological process of *cognitive defusion* corresponds to the dimension of cognition, the longing for coherence that has as its opposite and pathological response of cognitive fusion. Cognitive fusion is described when the individual is stuck in literalness and sees his thoughts as immutable truths, as a consequence the individual becomes fused to his mental contents and ends up organizing his behavior to correspond to the demands of this cognitive fusion. By not being able to see the larger context, he ends up becoming a prisoner of this pattern which distances him even more from both contact with the present moment and what is meaningful to him (Hayes et al., 2012a). Harris (2009) highlights thoughts and verbal processes with which the mind usually fuses. They are:

1. rules that the individual needs to comply with that distance him from his change (among them: I need, I must, I have to, I should, I can, or I can't);
2. reasons that justify and explain why change is impossible or unfeasible at this moment (for example, "I'm too busy"; "this is a genetic problem"; "I don't have money"; "it's too much for me"…);
3. judgments that bind them to literalness and bring suffering ("there's something wrong with me"; "life is not worth living"; "everyone is a liar"; "I am a failure");
4. moments from the past that produce ruminations about how good life was before and now it's no longer good with a focus on errors and failures and opportunities that were wasted ("if I had accepted that opportunity"; "my life was better decades ago and will never be the same again");
5. future situations that the individual worries excessively about (for example, what needs to be done later or when they have a better life);
6. self-evaluations that distance the individual from a meaningful life ("I am incapable of resisting and persisting"; "I am admired by no one"; "I am lazy") In fusion, thoughts dominate actions.

The defusion proposed by ACT advocates ways for the individual to detach from their thoughts and feelings, promoting a necessary distance between the person and their thoughts so that there is an awareness that they are just thoughts. That is, they respond to a way of thinking in context and do not fit all situations. It is an important psychoeducation in this process to understand that what the individual thinks is NOT the absolute truth, that they are just words and images that pass through their mind. Thus, the way they respond to these thoughts can be modified to promote psychological flexibility. Understanding how fusion occurs, the use of metaphors, experiential techniques, and mindfulness gives the individual new possibilities of action once they understand that thoughts do not direct their actions (Harris, 2009; Hayes et al., 2012a).

Some exercises proposed by Harris (2011) help the patient promote cognitive defusion. One of them, very simple and effective, consists of instructing the patient to bring a thought to consciousness and believe in it for 20 s. Example: "I will never be able to exercise". The next step will be to insert in front of this thought the phrase I am having the thought that… In the example above: "I am having the thought that I will never be able to exercise". At this moment the patient is instructed to observe what happens for a few seconds and then put in front of what they just thought the expression "I notice that…" then it would be "I notice that I am having the thought that I will never be able to exercise". At this stage, the patient is again invited to observe and perceive what happens. The goal of the exercise is to produce distance between the subject and the thought, and the insertion of the above phrases produces this effect.

The patient can do this with any difficult thought and this training is an excellent option to promote cognitive defusion. Another exercise proposed by the same author, widely used to promote defusion, is called the ridiculous voices technique in which the therapist asks the patient to think the disturbing thought as if it were being said with a funny or ridiculous voice like Goofy's; Donald Duck's; Scooby Doo's, right after thinking about it in their original voice. The patient can choose a character that they like or that makes sense to them or make a voice in "slow motion" articulating the syllables well or in a very high and strident tone in order to produce distance with the intention of promoting cognitive defusion. (Harris, 2011) In the same vein, Harris (2011) proposes the musicalization of thought, that is, asking the patient to put the thought into musical sounds. It can be their favorite samba, a lullaby, happy birthday, rock, among others. Any rhythm can be used to intone the difficult thought that will be sung in the chosen music. According to the author, putting the thought into a melody helps to realize that they are just words and, once again, increases the chance of promoting the desired distance in defusion.

Flexible Attention with the Present Moment

The psychological process of *attention to the present moment* corresponds to the dimension of attention. The opposite of this pathological response is being stuck and oriented to the past and/or the future. Being in the present moment stimulates the development of attention, free from criticism and judgments, and allows the individual to notice and observe the phenomena that occur around them with openness. Awareness of the present moment has its origin in mindfulness.

The present moment is all that the human being has because it is where life happens, and it is also where changes can occur. All ACT processes and contextual approaches are supported in the present moment. Therefore, many authors consider mindfulness a pillar for contextual approaches. The definition of the dimension of awareness to the present moment is sometimes confused with the definition of mindfulness which is "a flexible state of mind in which we are actively engaged in the present, perceiving new things and sensitive to context" (Langer, 2000) or "mindfulness is nothing more than concentration in the present moment, with an open mind and willing to understand what happens around and within you." (Snel, 2013).

The practice of mindfulness is often used to promote the process of paying attention to the present moment, and various exercises can be used as attention objects such as sounds, smells, touch, and breathing. The client is encouraged to focus attention on the chosen object and notice when disturbing thoughts and feelings arise. And in this case, the instruction is to observe the thoughts and feelings, thank them, and gently return attention to the exercise.

Various breathing exercises can be used as training tools for attention and increase of connection with the present moment. The "three-minute breathing space" exercise described by Pennan and Williams (2011) is a simple, efficient possibility with a duration of 3 min. The patient is instructed to adopt a comfortable position, stabilize in the position, and close their eyes. Then, they should slowly bring attention to the inner experience focusing on the following questions: what is my experience at this moment? What thoughts are on my mind? What feelings are here? What bodily sensations are present?

In the second stage, the patient will reorient their attention to focus on the physical sensations of breathing. Noticing and observing the abdominal movement, the movement of the nostrils and the path of the air entering and leaving the lungs using the breath to anchor in the present moment.

The third step of the exercise is the expansion of awareness around breathing including the perception of the body as a whole, posture, and facial expression. If the patient perceives sensations of discomfort or tension, they should direct attention to these sensations and inhale and exhale from these sensations in order to attenuate them and relax with the exhalation.

The goal is to increase attentional focus and train awareness to be in the present moment, and if by chance one's thoughts invade the exercise, the instruction is to observe, thank those thoughts, and gently return to the exercise. The authors suggest that this exercise be done at least three times a day to produce connection and take the patient further away from being stuck in the past or future, or from functioning in the mode of "automatic pilot" which means acting without awareness (Pennan & Williams, 2011; Williams & Penman, 2015).

Contextual Self/Observer Self

According to ACT, human suffering can come from arbitrary verbal relations and the vulnerability of a broader sense of self that can present mental disorders. Hayes states that there is an imbalance that needs to be worked on and suggests reducing the problem-solving mode of the mind. This mode prioritizes finding meaning and solutions for everyday experiences, in addition to making predictions and creating narratives which can contribute to the maintenance of suffering. Such behaviors project the individual into the past and future and distance them from experiences in the present moment. The solution to this lies in attentional flexibility which requires a distancing from the conceptual self, which leads the subject to distorted thinking and living imprisoned by their truths and critical constructions (Hayes, et al., 2011).

The psychologist's work in ACT is to instruct the patient to observe their posture and reactions to what happens in the context, helping to develop the observing self. The psychological process of the *contextual self* (or *observing self*) corresponds to the dimension of the self. The opposite for this pathological response is the conceptual self. In this way, it is believed that that clients will be able to transform their relationship with difficult thoughts and feelings (Araújo, et al., 2021).

There are several ways to work with the self as context with the aim of strengthening the patient's contact with perspective taking; among them are mindfulness techniques and the use of metaphors. An example of a brief mindfulness exercise that can be used at the beginning of a session to help promote perspective taking is to ask the client to observe the various sensations present at that moment, such as their breathing or the sounds of the environment. The practice continues with a brief centering exercise guided by the therapist as described below:

> "Now, as you observe these things, I want you to notice that you are observing these things. You are here now, aware of what you are aware of. If you're not sure, just wait for some time to notice a sensation or image...And notice that you are noticing... Don't try to hold onto this part and look at it—you would be looking from another place. Just touch this awareness lightly and notice that you are here, conscious, at this moment of your life... Now, I want you to think about all the things that can happen in our session today—we can examine what has been happening; what is difficult or pleasurable; what you fear or what you hope for; your pain and your values. Don't get tangled up in them now—just note that these issues are here and give them a moment to bubble around you... And then, I want you to imagine yourself many years from now looking back at this moment. You can see yourself sitting in this chair, aware of all the pains and fears and hopes and aspirations. Imagine that you have made progress and are now wiser. Don't overthink it but see if you can get in touch with this sense of awareness—of looking back at yourself now. Try to let go of any judgment and just focus on this person you see in a kind way in your consciousness. If this could really happen, what advice would you give yourself about how to engage in this session we are about to begin? Don't answer quickly... just put yourself inside this question for a few moments... See if there is anything you could tell yourself if this could really happen. If there is, just note what it is. See if you can connect with a caring and self-compassionate self. Do you have anything to say? Connect with this message, almost as if you were about to express it out loud. Now, return inside your body... Imagine where I am. And, when you are ready to start, just open your eyes and use the next few minutes to write down the message that came to your mind." (Hayes et al., 2021, pp. 183)

The aim of this practice and the psychologist's other choices in working with the dimensions of the self are related to helping the patient establish greater perspective taking. Metaphors are also used abundantly at this time; they are particularly useful to highlight the differences between context and content of consciousness.

The clinician should encourage the patient to observe and not seek immediate solutions. That is, the therapist's role is to help the client make direct contact with the experience of consciousness, without analysis and interpretations. In other words, the therapist should help the individual experience knowledge that goes beyond the verbal.

Values

The psychological process of values corresponds to the dimension of motivation, the longing for meaning and purpose in life. The opposite pathological response is the lack of clarity of values. The *values* in ACT, are the heart of human sense and purpose, as they provide a constructive, consistent direction and support the process of behavioral flexibility. For ACT, from the moment actions are guided by values, the individual becomes willing, open, and motivated to walk towards a life with meaning.

That being said, values need to be the consequences of free choices, without judgment. The individual will reflect on what is important to him and this will help him develop a process of appreciation that should guide his actions even after the end of therapy. Another important point in the construction of values is the understanding that they are not feelings, for example, feeling love for a person is different from valuing a life with love. Values are choices, not feelings (Hayes et al., 2012b).

One of the most powerful exercises of ACT that provides tools for the construction of values during the therapeutic process is called What Do You Want Your Life to Mean? The therapist asks the patient to close their eyes and relax for a few minutes in order to clear their mind of everything that is in it at that moment. (This can last about 2–3 min.) Then, the patient is guided to imagine that, by some whim of fate, they died, but managed to attend their own funeral in spirit. With this, the patient will be observing and listening to the tribute made by their spouse, their children, their friends, the people they worked with, etc. They are asked to just imagine the situation and emotionally place themselves in the scene. After that, they are guided to visualize how they would like these people who were part of their life to remember them. The therapist asks questions like "what would you like your wife to say about you as a husband?" The patient is encouraged to verbalize. (Here the therapist pauses and lets the client speak.) This work continues with the other people the patient relates to, for example, how they would like their children to remember them as a father and their colleagues at work.

It is important that they are encouraged to say what they would like, even if in reality they have not lived according to what they would like. After the patient verbalizes how they would like all the significant people in their life to remember them, the therapist helps the client to reorient to the session, for example: "When you are ready, simply open your eyes". An alternative to this experience could be to ask the client to write a small epitaph on an imaginary tombstone, or to think about a surprise video prepared by close people to celebrate a milestone birthday. Often, this exercise reveals how incompatible the client's values are with their current actions.

In therapy, patients are encouraged through effective conversations to get in touch with their values and declare them explicitly. The process of making very close experiential contact with one's own values is one of the most intense and intimate clinical experiences in ACT. It brings vitality, a sense of choice, orientation to the present moment, and a willingness to be vulnerable (Luoma et al., 2022). A final benefit of value construction is that it can trigger a perception that life is happening now and not somewhere in the future.

More objectively, there is a list of value domains that can be personalized with each client (table below). It is important to highlight the importance of differentiating values from goals, values are directions and goals have an end in themselves. The work with value domains begins in the session and the patient is encouraged to continue at home. The patient is instructed to write "nothing" when they do not identify with a certain value. It is important to emphasize that values are socially constructed and individually chosen.

- Family relationships (other than marriage or parenthood)
- Marriage/partnership/intimate relationships
- Parenthood (motherhood/fatherhood)
- Friendships/social relationships
- Career/employment
- Education/training/personal growth and development
- Recreation/fun
- Spirituality
- Community life
- Health/Physical Self-Care
- Environment/Sustainability
- Art/Aesthetics

One of the goals of working with values is to generate committed actions that are consistent with the person's values. As a rule, therapists should spend considerable time in sessions understanding the psychological valence of values before moving on to discussions about commitment action. Essentially, the therapist needs to understand the psychological implications of getting the client to start acting in a valued domain. How is this action associated with the client's story about themselves? What are the potential sources of fusion if the client starts making moves in this area? In some situations, the therapist should invite the patient to contemplate more rather than seek actions. This experiential experience in itself has much more value than certain attitudes and problem-solving pursuits.

Commitment or Committed Actions

The psychological process of commitment corresponds to the dimension of behavior, and the longing for competence has impulsivity and avoidance as its pathological response. It can be said that at this stage of treatment the patient is invited to put into practice the changes they wish to make in their life, or changes that are important to them to lead a valuable life (Harris, 2011; Saban, 2015).

After identifying the values, the therapist helps the client create contingencies that allow them to experience their values or that help them get closer to them (Wilson et al., 2012). Behavioral changes revolve around chosen values, while opening up space for new experiences.

Committed action includes specific attitudes at certain times, while value-based action involves freely chosen and verbally constructed qualities of continuous action. Value-based actions are those that are deliberately conceived by the individual to bring them closer to a particular value and are strongly reinforced.

Willingness and commitment help patients go through difficult situations by understanding that they are linked to their values. At the same time, it frees the patient from painful relationships driven by fear. Another important point is that commitment actions are never perfect or constant, but always intentional. The patient is strongly encouraged to act towards value action. This conceptualization and intervention proposal in mind, the premise of ACT is not to make the individual free from suffering, but rather to learn more adaptive and flexible repertoires to deal with their afflictions and move in the direction of what is important to them (Wilson et al., 2012). At this point, once again the use of metaphors is encouraged. The intention is for the patient to understand that availability, choice, valuation, actions, and barriers are part of a powerful life.

The Gardening metaphor is among the most used metaphors to emphasize how conscious choice can allow the individual to stay on a fixed course in the face of difficult, provocative, or confusing feedback.

"Imagine that you chose a place to make a garden. You worked the soil, planted the seeds, and waited for them to sprout. In the meantime, you started to notice a place across the street that also seemed good—maybe even better. So, you pulled up your vegetables, crossed the street, and made another garden there. After that, you noticed another place that seemed even better. Values are like the place where you make your garden. You can grow some things very quickly, but some things require time and dedication. So, the question is: 'Do you want to have your livelihood based on lettuce or do you want to live off something more substantial—potatoes, beets, or something similar?'. You can't figure out how things work in gardens when you have to put up stakes repeatedly. Now, of course, if you stay in the same place, you will start to notice its imperfections. Maybe the soil isn't as level as it seemed when you started, or the water has to be transported a long distance. Some things you plant may give the impression that they take a lifetime to sprout. In moments like these, your mind will tell you that 'you should have planted somewhere else', 'this probably will never work', 'it was foolish of you to think you could grow anything here', etc. The choice to plant here allows you to water, pull, and weed even when these thoughts and feelings arise. You are building a broader pattern. You are not just watering—you are watering your garden. You are not just digging; you are digging your garden." (pp. 266; Hayes et al., 2021). This metaphor is a rich way to guide clients towards more committed actions. For example, if the patient values self-care, this metaphor can encourage them to be more active in this area. Walking in the morning can, in certain aspects, be like weeding, however, it is important to make clear that it is not about the walk itself. It is the connection with what he considers self-care in a broader sense—that is, taking care of oneself or the garden is what gives meaning to these individual moments of action and gives him the power to lead to broader patterns of value-based behavior.

The ACT-Matrix diagram was developed by Kevin Polk, Mark Webster, and Jerold Hambright to facilitate clinical practice in pursuit of psychological flexibility (Polk & Schoendorff, 2014). According to Polk et al. (2016) the Matrix is a didactic and playful way to organize the psychological processes of ACT and brings greater awareness of the elements of the context that influence the patient's behavior. He also considers the Matrix a metaphor that promotes the "deliteralization" of psychological content allowing the patient to see in perspective and behind the linguistic contents that perpetuate inflexibility.

In practice, the Matrix diagram provides contextual clues through questions that evoke specific responses that affect the client's behavior. The diagram consists of a graph with four quadrants in which the intersection of these quadrants is the place where the client is observing. The top of the diagram reflects external observation using the senses and the bottom the internal observation of what is going on in the mind. The right side of the Matrix brings the patient closer to what is important to him, and the left side moves the patient away from what is important to him. The first quadrant represents avoidance behaviors, the second commitment or approach behaviors, the quadrant below represents what or who is important to the patient and the last quadrant the internal obstacles.

Polk et al. (2016) consider that some questions are asked to the client when filling out the diagram. The authors suggest that therapists start with the quadrant of what is important to the patient and the question is: "Who or what is important to you?" This quadrant includes things, people, goals that patients want to achieve to get closer to what is important to them. The next quadrant to be filled is the internal obstacles and the question is "What are your internal obstacles that appear on the way?" This quadrant includes thoughts, emotions, physical reactions that occur when the person feels they are distancing themselves from values and/or feeling in suffering. It is important that the patient understands that approaching their values will make him face obstacles. The next quadrant to be filled is avoidance behaviors and the central question is: "What do you do when you feel that you are suffering and still remain suffering?" "What do you do in the face of emotion/thought or physical reaction that moves you away from what is good for you?" And in the last quadrant to be filled, the approach behaviors, the patient answers the questions: "What behaviors do you have that bring you closer to what is important to you?" "Instead of having a flight/avoidance behavior what can you do to get closer to your

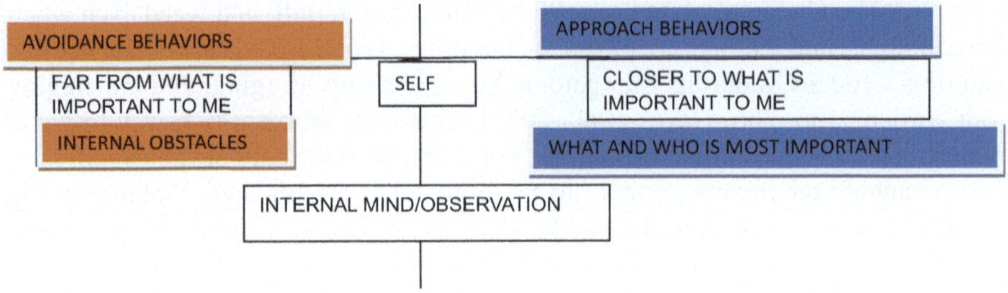

Fig. 8.2 Five senses of internal observations

values?" And last but not least, the observer-self is reinforced in the center of the diagram and the patient is invited to notice this with the question: "Who can perceive this?" In this way, the patient is trained for perspective-taking, where they can choose behaviors aligned with their values (Polk et al., 2016). Figure 8.2 represents the five senses of internal observations.

Clinical Case

M., 51 years old, is the head nurse of a neonatal ICU in a large city in a highly reputable hospital network that serves private patients in the south zone of the city. She seeks therapy at the insistence of the unit's chief doctors, as they claim she is struggling to cope with the necessary adaptations to the new functioning of the unit. As they greatly appreciate her and her 30 years of dedicated service, they decide to pay for her therapy so she can make the changes she needs. M. heads the neonatal intensive care unit with 8 beds and almost 20 nursing technicians, in addition to providing support to doctors and families. A very challenging, yet very rewarding job, as the client herself reports. According to the client, the problem began when the hospital network was sold to a large national chain and with the sale came many changes not only in the organization of work, but also in the administrative part that she was not used to doing in the other hospital network. The new assignments have raised concerns of complaints, criticism, and "unprofessional" attitudes according to the coordinating doctors of the service. She vents and says that she doesn't understand spreadsheets, but rather patients and care. And with the new administration, she is responsible for spreadsheets that she is not interested in learning to fill out, in addition to creating confusion to accept any change. M. has always been hardworking and a very attentive and obedient daughter, however, her parents described her as very headstrong and stubborn. She needed to understand the reasons for things before she would do something new or that was not in her repertoire. She reports that she never had trouble studying and doing her school tasks and that she was always an excellent student and already left nursing school employed. Her level of dedication to work is maximum and because of this, she is proud to be the head nurse of such a renowned institution. M. got married at 30, but her marriage did not survive the shifts and the extra work hours she voluntarily took on to be recognized for her excellence. After 3 years trying to maintain the marriage, M. returned to her parents' house where she lives to this day with her cat and parakeet. She reports that she prefers the peace of living alone with her pets to having to share space with someone who will question her choices and stress her out.

The client's complaint is her mood swings throughout the day, constant irritability, symptoms of anxiety linked to the new assignments from the changes at work, difficulty adapting to some rules that do not make sense to her, and a need to be respected. The patient reports having had panic attacks throughout her life in specific situations, such as after her father's death; when she was responding to an administrative process for having insulted a former hospital director; when she feels her job is at risk. She reports that she has always had a high level of concern and anxiety about everything. She has been diagnosed with obsessive-compulsive disorder for liking things "perfect" and making many checklists and verifications, but has never undergone psychiatric or psychological treatment.

Ever since the hospital was bought by the new network, she feels insecure, like a failure, as she invested everything in her profession and now feels that she needs to prove herself again and feels unequipped to deal with the new context. In the evaluation of psychological dimensions we can highlight: in the dimension of self, the patient is stuck in the conceptual self when she does not feel like herself and despairs when she does not recognize herself; in the dimension of affect, the patient is in experiential avoidance of the administrative work she needs to develop and avoids in every way this contact and all the unpleasant feelings that this evokes; in the dimension of cognition, she is fused to the thought that she invested everything in work to get where she is and it is not fair "to have to start everything from scratch"; in the attention dimension, she projects catastrophic scenarios in which she will be humiliated and fired from her job; in the motivation dimension, she lacks clarity about her values and focuses on trying to maintain subjective control, not reporting the meaning of work and affective relationships.

Finally, in the behavior dimension, she spends most of her time reacting aggressively to the attempts of assistance that both her bosses and coworkers offer. M. reports various situations where it is clear that she fears being seen as someone who cannot handle new functions and her inflexibility causes adaptation problems to the new rules.

Below is the Matrix made with the patient, which illustrates these situations with the aim of increasing awareness of the process, facilitating defusion, and building the observing self. She keeps ruminating predictions that she will lose her job; she doesn't handle administrative spreadsheets; she avoids meetings with bosses and those about demands; she increases the demands and control over the team; she wants to be more loving and calmer with the team; she wants to try to understand the spreadsheets with openness and goodwill; she wants to ask for help and accept help when offered; she wants to participate in meetings and ask for training to develop. "I will have to prove that I am good again" and "It's not fair that I have to do administrative work at this stage of the game" with feelings of failure, anger, sadness, fear, and inadequacy. She wants to be recognized for her value and work;

Have the trust of doctors and families; Be recognized as a reference by her team; Her cat and parakeet; Her nieces.

The construction of the Matrix along with M helped the patient to increase awareness about her psychological processes and served as a starting point for clinical intervention. M.'s biggest challenge was to defuse from the thoughts that she "would have to start from scratch" and that "it was not fair to have to do the administrative spreadsheets". And this was the starting point of therapy.

Along with this important defusion, the client was invited to reduce the control and demands she made on her work team, as the harsh and rude demands only served to isolate her from people and were more a way of avoiding the administrative work, she couldn't handle than effectively a demand for greater team productivity.

Thus, gradually, she would be able to accept her condition and do something in the direction of understanding the new job, which was important to the client, and, for example, allow herself to ask for and accept help to deal with the new tasks she didn't even know where to start. To defuse, colorful post-it labels were used with various thoughts that paralyzed her and phrases were inserted like "I notice that I'm having the thought that…" and the patient was saying the phrases with a very deep voice as if she were a character and then with a very high voice producing an important observation distance.

Several mindfulness exercises were used so that they could be incorporated into her daily life in order for her to connect with actions committed to her values that were organized in therapy. Exploring the sensory experience of coffee as a mindfulness exercise helped her a lot to produce a cut-off line with behaviors that distanced her from what was important and connected her with behaviors that brought her closer to what is important, as the patient had a loving relationship with coffee and the experience was very positive.

Gradually, M defused from the thoughts that were obstacles and managed to engage in training and reconnected with the M. who loved to study and learn and challenged herself to understand what she needed for her new tasks. From this point, M started creating goals with "acceptance, trust, and commitment to their values and discovering new values such as love for learning and interest in trying new things.

Today, M. has regained the admiration of her team and bosses and continues to learn and challenge herself, understanding well the role of Mindfulness exercises and their psychological dimensions that have contributed to a healthier and more flexible M.

Conclusion

In conclusion, ACT strives to foster psychological flexibility, helping individuals accept their thoughts and emotions while guiding them toward committed actions aligned with their values. ACT approaches on accepting one's thoughts and feelings while committing to personal values. Individuals can cultivate a more compassionate relationships with their own thoughts and emotions. The ultimate goal is to promote a rich and meaningful life by navigating challenges with resilience and mindfulness.

References

Araújo, R. et al. (2021) *Guia Teórico- Pratico de Terapias Cognitivo-Comportamentais para os Transtornos do Exagero* (pp. 212–280). Ed. Sinopsys.

Fletcher, L., & Hayes, S. C. (2005). Relational frame theory, acceptance and commitment therapy, and a functional analytic definition of mindfulness. *Journal of Rational- Emotive & Cognitive-Behavior Therapy, 23*(4), 315–336. https://doi.org/10.1007/s10942-005-0017-7

Harris, R. (2009). *ACT made simple: An easy-to-read primer on acceptance and commitment therapy*. New Harbinger.

Harris, R. (2011). *The confidence gap: A guide to overcoming fear and self-doubt*. Trumpeter Books.

Hayes, S. C. (2004). Acceptance and commitment therapy and the new behavior therapies: Mindfulness, acceptance and relationship. In S. C. Hayes, V. M. Follette, S. C. Hayes, J. B. Luoma, F. W. Bond, A. Masuda, & J. Lillis. (2006, January). Acceptance and commitment therapy: Model, processes and outcomes. *Behaviour Research and Therapy, 44*(1), 1–25. https://doi.org/10.1016/j.brat.2005.06.006. PMID: 16300724.

Hayes, S., Luoma, J., Bond, F., Masuda, A., & Lillis, J. (2006). Acceptance and commitment therapy: Model, process and outcomes. *Behaviour Research and Therapy, 44*(1), 1–25

Hayes, S., Strosahl, K., & Wilson, K. (1999, 2012). *Acceptance and commitment therapy: The process and practice of mindful change*. Guilford Publications.

Hayes, S. C., Follette, V. M., & Linehan, M. M. (Eds.). (2011). *Mindfulness and acceptance: Expanding the cognitive behavioral tradition* (pp. 1–29). Guilford Publications.

Hayes, S. C., Pistorello, J., & Levin, M. E. (2012a). Acceptance and commitment therapy as a unified model of behavior change. *The Counseling Psychologist, 40*(7), 976–1002. https://doi.org/10.1177/0011000012460836

Hayes, S., Strosahl, K., & Wilson, K. (2012b). *Acceptance and commitment therapy: the process and practice of mindful change 2nd ed.* Guilford Press

Langer, E. J. (2000). Mindful learning. *Current Directions in Psychological Science, 9*(6), 220–223. https://doi.org/10.1111/1467-8721.00099

Lucena-Santos, P., Cunha, M. A., & Pinto-Gouveia, J. A. (2021). *Terapia de Aceitação e Compromisso*. Ed Sinopsys.

Luoma, J. B., Hayes, S. C., & Walser, R. D. (2022). *Aprendendo a ACT: Manual de habilidades da terapia de aceitação e compromisso para terapeutas*. Sinopsys Editora.

Pennan, D., Williams, M. (2011) Mindfulness: A Practical Guide to Finding Peace in a Frantic World. Piatkus Books.

Polk, K., & Schoendorff, B. (2014). *The ACT—MATRIX a new approach to building psychological flexibility across settings & populations*. New Harbinger.

Polk, K. L., Schoendorff, B., Webster, M., & Olaz, F. O. (2016). *The essential guide to the ACT matrix: A step-by-step approach to using the ACT matrix model in clinical practice*. New Harbinger.

Saban, M. (2015). *Introdução a Terapia de Aceitação e Compromisso*. Ed. Artesã.

Snel, E. (2013). *Sitting still like a frog: Mindfulness exercises for kids (and their parents)*. Shambhala Publications, Incorporated.

Wilson, K., Schnetzer, L., Flynn, M., & Kurz, A. (2012). Acceptance and commitment therapy for addictions. In S. Hayes & M. Lewin (Eds), *Mindfulness & acceptance for addictive behaviors: applying contextual CBT to substance abuse & behaviors addictions* (pp27–68). Context Press.

Williams, M., Penman, D. (2015). Atenção Plena: como encontrar a paz em um mundo frenético Rio de Janeiro: Sextante.

Chapter 9
Metacognitive Therapy (MCT): Transdiagnostic Approach to Improve Cognitive Functioning, Problem-Solving, and Emotional Well-Being

Heitor P. Hirata

Introduction

The prefix "meta" comes from Greek and means transcendence within critical reflection on something, while cognition refers to thoughts or cognitive processes (Moses & Baird, 2001; Flavell, 1979). While CBT emphasizes the modification of the content of cognitions, MCT assists in changing the way individuals think (Wells, 2009). Thus, metacognition refers to reflection directed at thoughts. The term is not coined from Wells' work. Flavell (1979) already pointed out metacognition as the ability of children to perceive the occurrence of the learning process. For an individual to notice that he knows something, he needs to perceive what is happening in his mind and even ask himself questions to monitor his degree of understanding. For example, when reading this text, the reader may ask himself: "am I understanding this"? If so, he moves on; otherwise, he reads again. This monitoring of understanding about an object of knowledge is also considered metacognition and the roots of the term go back to this field.

Attention and Emotion as Interconnected Elements

Wells and Matthews (1994) pointed out several studies that show how the attentional process interferes with emotions. Indeed, from a clinical perspective, it can be seen that many of the problems brought by patients are related to attentional focus directed at threats. This can occur both in the case of a psychiatric disorder such as generalized anxiety disorder (GAD), obsessive-compulsive disorder (OCD), depression; as well as in individuals without a diagnosis.

H. P. Hirata (✉)
Rio de Janeiro, RJ, Brazil

A. C. Ornelas (ed.), *Transdiagnostic Approaches in Cognitive Behavioral Therapy*, https://doi.org/10.1007/978-3-031-63494-9_9

Complaints that fall within the scope of "emotional dysregulation" are often permeated with problems in attentional biases. For example: a patient who complains of "impulsivity" and "excessive anger" probably unknowingly directs his attention to external and internal stimuli that amplify this emotion, increasing the chances of behaviors that cause problems for him in his environment. Another example is jealousy. People who usually bring this type of complaint often focus their attention on stimuli that intensify this emotion.

A patient may report that he is always looking at his girlfriend's cell phone screen when it lights up, as his attention is always focused on the possibilities of betrayal. In a traditional cognitive-behavioral approach (Beck, 1976), the evidence that he is being cheated on would be addressed. Within a metacognitive approach, the focus is on how problematic it is for the client to have rigid attentional biases that continually turn to signs of "betrayal" and also to thoughts related to this subject. Thus, it can be understood that working with attention, which is not restricted to Metacognitive Therapy, is an important feature of this approach, being a transdiagnostic element, as it permeates various complaints whether they are related to a diagnosis or not.

Central Concepts of Metacognitive Therapy

To properly understand this approach, some essential concepts need to be elucidated. They are:

1. Self-Regulatory Executive Function Model (S-REF)
2. Attentional Cognitive Syndrome (SCA)
3. Metacognitive beliefs

Self-Regulatory Executive Function Model (S-REF)

The S-REF model was presented by Wells and Matthews (1994) and consists of an explanatory model about the operation of cognition levels. The authors suggest three levels: (1) automatic processing level; (2) online processing level and (3) stored knowledge level. The automatic processing level refers to all cognitive content (thoughts) that passes through consciousness. Much of this volume will not even be noticed by the individual, as tens of thousands of intrusive thoughts can arise, but there is no possibility of paying attention to all of them. Some of these thoughts go to level 2, online processing, which involves the investment of attentional resources. At this level, the thoughts that receive attention can contribute to the mobilization of emotional resources. Then level 3, the stored knowledge, involves the activation of metacognitive beliefs, which will be addressed shortly.

Figure 9.1 illustrates the S-REF model in a playful way to contribute to the elucidation of the concepts.

The illustration contains the playful idea of the "thought-producing factory". It's as if we had a device that continuously produces thoughts incessantly in large volumes. Much of this production is not even perceived and is simply discarded. A small part receives the focus of attention (symbolized by the ghost). This small portion of cognition is the target of attention and can take the form of cognitive processes such as worry or rumination, for example. This, in turn, will bring up unpleasant emotions with which patients have difficulty managing and, thus, may end up emitting coping behaviors that often bring harmful consequences to their lives.

Attentional Cognitive Syndrome (SCA)

According to the perspective of the S-REF model and the theory that underpins MCT, all psychological disorders are permeated by a specific style of thought and ways of relating to aversive intrusive thoughts (Wells, 2009). This style is called attentional cognitive syndrome, which refers to a persistent allocation of attention in thought that takes the form of worry, rumination, and focus on threats (Fisher & Wells, 2009).

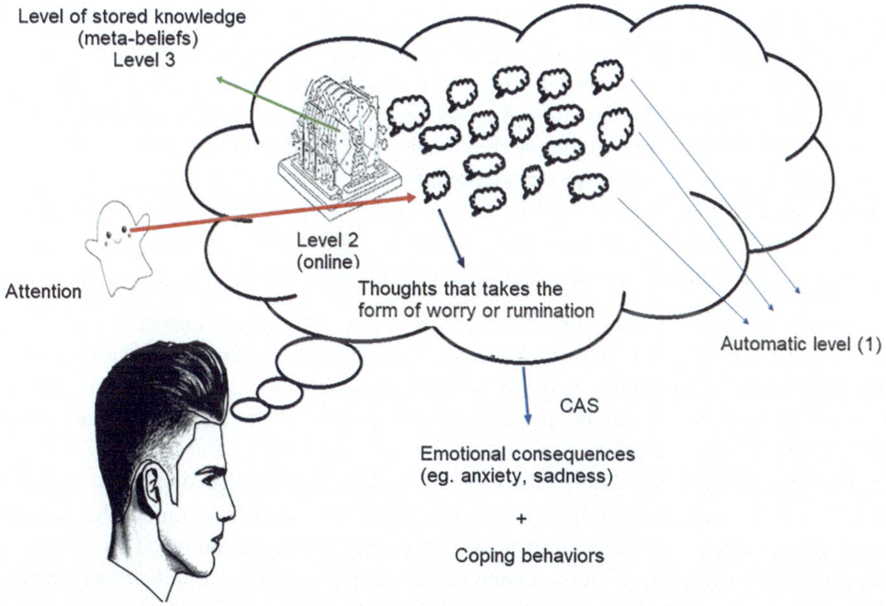

Fig. 9.1 Self-Regulatory Executive Function Model (S-REF model), based on Wells (2009). (Source: Author's file)

The SCA is the product of attention focused on trigger thoughts (produced by the machine), which take the form of worry or rumination. The following clinical dialogue illustrates the SCA process.

Therapist: So, Maria, you said there was something that had bothered you throughout this week. Do you want to talk about it?
Maria: Yes. I've been thinking too much! Especially when it's time to sleep. I toss and turn in bed, try to stop thinking, but I can't. I think I'm going crazy.
Therapist: I see. Why don't you tell me what you've been thinking about?
Maria: I keep thinking about how much I have to do, and I end up not getting anything done. I also think about the ridiculous role I play every time I fail to do something important and have to communicate that to others. There's so much that I can't even start sometimes…
Therapist: Right, so you're overwhelmed and when you think you have to take care of a new task, you immediately have a thought that you won't be able to handle this task?
Maria: That's right.
Therapist: And then what comes next?
Maria: I think others will see me as irresponsible, that they will never trust me again.
Therapist: And what comes next?
Maria: That I will be isolated professionally and personally, I will end up alone.
Therapist: And then…
Maria: And then I will be ruined!
Therapist: How does that make you feel?
Maria: More restless, anxious.
Therapist: Maria, what if we consider that part of your problem comes from how much you end up "clinging" to the initial thoughts that arise? For example: just now you said that the first thought you had was "I have a lot to do, and I can't handle anything". Do you realize that what you started thinking from this thought generated more thoughts and more anxiety?
Maria: Yes, I realize.
Therapist: Well then, we can say that you entered a process of worry, generated by the excessive attention you directed to this initial thought.

In Maria's case, the SCA occurred from the moment the initial thought "I have a lot to do, and I can't handle anything" became the focus of attention and from it, other thoughts arose, generating a spiral of new thoughts and unpleasant emotions. Maria's SCA process can be illustrated in Fig. 9.2, from an analogy with the Matryoshka, or Russian doll.

The Matryoshka model helps the patient to notice the step-by-step process of the SCA. In this case, the attentional process interferes with how much the person "opens more dolls", giving room for the emergence of new thoughts. Thus, there is the possibility of opening many Matryoshkas even beyond the smallest one. When this point is reached, the suffering is probably greatly amplified. The "simple" noticing that the SCA process is occurring already helps patients to realize that it

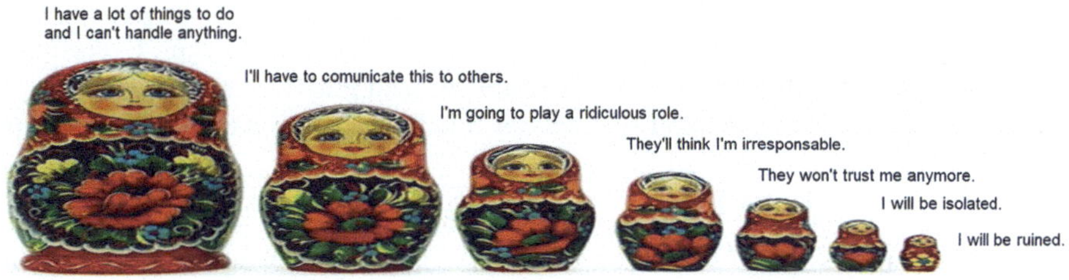

Fig. 9.2 Illustration of the SCA model from the Matryoshka model. (Source: Author's file)

can be interrupted. However, often they do not know how. At this point, MCT techniques can help, which will be discussed later.

Metacognitive Beliefs

Level 3 of Fig. 9.1 refers to metacognitive beliefs, a central concept of MCT. To address this aspect, it is important first to make a distinction between positive and negative beliefs about cognitive processes. To facilitate understanding, this text will only address worry and rumination.

Every individual, starting in childhood and continuing throughout their life learns ways to worry or ruminate. Some family environments facilitate the SCA process. For example, parents who react with a startle every time an accident occurs, tend to cause a startle reaction in children every time something unexpected happens. The following clinical vignette illustrates this:

Jorge: This week I had a feeling of being scared at various moments.

Therapist: Can you identify any event that is behind this feeling?

Jorge: I'm not exactly sure, but this week was atypical, many different things happened. I sent an important project by mail to a company I work for, and it took much longer than expected to arrive. I had to arrange another document and send it by courier. Also, the power went out a few times at my house and my daughter got very sick.

Therapist: These were unforeseen events, certainly. What catches my attention is that you said you were scared and not frustrated. What makes you think you were scared?

Jorge: Because I had a feeling of fright, as if I had to prepare for something much worse. I thought the project wouldn't arrive on time, that the power wouldn't come back on soon and I wouldn't be able to do anything, that I would have to take my daughter to the doctor, and it could be something worse!

Therapist: I notice that in the face of unforeseen events you had thoughts that sounded quite threatening to you. Has this always happened this way for you?

Jorge: I remember my parents always being scared or reactive to anything that deviated from the expected. As you said, it wasn't just frustration. It was a real scare.

If a glass broke it was a drama, if someone got sick it was very dangerous, if it rained you couldn't leave the house because an accident might occur. Everything was a reason for a big drama. Even a simple broken glass!

Therapist: Noticing this, do you realize that this has become part of your way of reacting to situations as well?

Jorge: Certainly. And in a way, deep down I think this kind of thinking can protect me.

Jorge's story refers to the formation of positive beliefs about worry ("worry can protect me"), which is based on his history with parents who were always startled by unforeseen events. Tables 9.1 and 9.2 exemplify other types of metacognitive beliefs.

Positive and negative beliefs about worries constitute, therefore, metacognitive beliefs. These, when activated, bias attentional resources to focus on specific thoughts, giving rise to SCA, as illustrated in Fig. 9.1.

Metacognitive Therapy Techniques

MCT has some specific techniques of the approach that can be useful for managing problems related to SCA. In this chapter, five will be mentioned:

1. Techniques of detached mindfulness (DM)
2. Attention training (AT)
3. Socratic dialogue focused on metacognition
4. Metacognition-based exposure
5. Personification of cognitive processes

Table 9.1 Positive beliefs about worries and ruminations

Worries	Ruminations
"Worries help me deal with problems."	"Rumination helps me understand problems."
"If I worry, I will be prepared for problems."	"If I analyze why I am feeling this way, I will find answers."
"Worries keep me safe."	"Ruminating helps me understand my depression."
"Worries help me do things well."	"Rumination helps me solve problems."
"Something bad could happen if I don't worry."	"Ruminating I will be trying to find ways out of depression."
"Worry helps me solve problems."	
"Worrying keeps people I love safe."	

Table 9.2 Negative beliefs about worries and ruminations

Worries	Ruminations
"I will go crazy with this worry." "If I don't control my worry, it will control me."	I can't control my depressive thoughts My depressive thoughts control me
"Worry puts my body under stress."	My depressive thoughts are a sign that I am losing my mind
"My worry is uncontrollable."	I am abnormal because I am thinking like that
"Worry can cause me harm."	My rumination is uncontrollable

Source: Adapted from Wells (2009)

Techniques of Detached Mindfulness (DM)

Detached Mindfulness, according to Wells (2006), is the antithesis of SCA. It consists of a style of disengagement from cognitive processes such as worry and rumination. The main goal of this technique is to shift the patient from object mode (non-differentiation of thought and reality) to metacognitive processing mode (awareness of thought as a mind event). Wells (2006) points out five main characteristics of DM: (1) meta-awareness, or awareness of thoughts; (2) cognitive decentering—understanding thoughts as events and not facts; (3) attentional disengagement, that is, not anchoring attention in an event; (4) low conceptual processing, that is, less analytical thinking and evaluation of the meanings of events and (5) reduction of goal-oriented coping—removal or avoidance of threat is not priority. DM work in the clinic is done through some metaphors, such as the tiger task, the cloud metaphor, and the train metaphor. For more details, see Wells (2009).

Attention Training (AT)

Attention training is a technique of MCT that aims to help the patient develop attentional flexibility. The original proposal by Wells (2009) is made from various simultaneous sounds arranged in the environment. At first, the patient should focus on only one of the sounds, then he should change the attentional direction to another sound and so on until all the sounds are completed. After this stage, the therapist instructs the person to pay attention to all the sounds in the environment simultaneously and to make a quick change in focus on each sound. The exercise should start with fewer sounds and, gradually, add new stimuli.

Socratic Dialogue Focused on Metacognition

Just as in traditional Cognitive Therapy where the Socratic dialogue is worked on, in MCT this technique is also used. However, the goal is different. While in CBT the aim is to delve into the content of cognitions in order to restructure distorted thought patterns (Beck, 1976), in MCT this technique is used to stop the SCA and challenge metacognitive beliefs (Wells, 2009).

The clinical dialogue below exemplifies the technique within the context of MCT:

Therapist: Anna, tell me a little about your week.

Anna: This week I had many depressive thoughts, I felt very down. I didn't feel like doing absolutely anything. In fact, today I almost didn't come to therapy.

Therapist: What kinds of depressive thoughts are these?

Anna: The usual ones… I thought that nothing is going right in my life, that there is no point in continuing to do what I do and that I can't find a new direction (rumination).

Therapist: Stopping to think about these thoughts that often come up in your head is what we call rumination. How much do you notice that rumination helps in these situations?

Anna: Of course it doesn't help! I get sadder and sadder, but I can't stop ruminating (negative belief about rumination: "rumination is uncontrollable").

Therapist: Have there been times when you were able to notice a trigger thought and it didn't become a rumination?

Anna: I think so. But I can't do that all the time.

Therapist: So, would it be correct to say that rumination is not uncontrollable? Perhaps the initial intrusive thought is yes, uncontrollable. But remember the Matryoshka (Fig. 9.2)? If you take one thought out of the other, it becomes rumination and it does depend on our attention.

Anna: But what to do then?

Therapist: We can go back to the exercises we discussed before about how to flex our attention.

In the dialogue above, it can be seen that Anna initially was ruminating without realizing the process and this was making her hopeless. The therapist's intervention, using Socratic dialogue focused on metacognition, was aimed at (1) identifying the ruminative process itself; (2) identifying the negative belief about rumination and (3) working to restructure the meta belief and flexible attention.

Metacognition-Based Exposure

Just like the Socratic dialogue, exposures also have a different objective in MCT compared to traditional CBT (Wells, 2009). While in CBT the intention is to foster the habituation mechanism, in MCT the idea is to challenge positive and/or negative beliefs about cognitive processes. For example: a patient with excessive unproductive worries (those that are not aimed at solving a problem and lead nowhere) may consider that worries are really useful (positive belief about worry). In this case, he can be challenged to point out situations where it actually helped, as illustrated by the dialogue below.

Therapist: So, Carlos, you told me that you have many worries going through your head throughout this week. Want to tell me a little more about them?
Carlos: Yes, I've been worrying quite a lot lately about everything: work, my family, my health.
Therapist: And have you noticed whether or not worrying about all this has helped?
Carlos: Well, what a silly question! Of course, worrying helps! I've worried a lot throughout my entire life, and stayed alert to possible unforeseen events, and here I am, alive!
Therapist: No doubt, worry can help. We have already talked about how worries can be divided between those that help (productive) and those that do not help (unproductive). It seems that you have identified several situations where worry was productive. But were all these that you had throughout the week really useful?
Carlos: Well, I don't know… Maybe not.
Therapist: Not EVERY worry is going to help. Let's do an exercise here. Can you think of something that is afflicting you at this exact moment in your life, but that does not depend on a practical resolution? Something that you have to wait and see what happens.
Carlos: Yes. I had some tests done about 3 weeks ago. The results come out at the end of this week, and I will talk to the doctor.
Therapist: Right. You understand that you have no control whatsoever about the results of the tests. What you could do, was to go to the doctor and take the tests, and you have already done that.
Carlos: That's right, it was within my control.
Therapist: So now try to worry with all intensity about the results of the test. Think about everything that can happen. I'll set a timer for a minute.
After a minute
Carlos: I got more anxious. I notice my heart beating.
Therapist: Right, that makes sense since you imagined quite unpleasant scenarios. At the same time, I would like to reflect here with you. Can this time that you spent worrying actually change anything about the results of the tests?
Carlos: Of course not!
Therapist: So, this is the point. Not all worries are useful (challenge to the positive belief about worry). Some, like this one from the exercise you just did, are not only useless but increase your suffering.

In the same way that this dialogue challenged the positive beliefs about worry, it is possible to challenge other types of beliefs (positive or negative) aimed at other cognitive processes, such as rumination, threat monitoring, obsessive thoughts, among others.

Personification of Cognitive Processes

The personification of cognitive processes involves giving a name to worry, rumination, obsessive thoughts, or other processes. The idea is to create a distance between the patient and their thoughts, putting them into perspective and favoring processing in a metacognitive mode.

Hirata and Gabriel (2017) developed a methodology that personifies cognitive processes such as worry, rumination, and obsessive thoughts. Initially, the proposal was directed towards children, but it can easily be adapted for other age groups. The proposal culminated in a children's book (Hirata & Gabriel, 2018).

As worry and rumination are processes that occur with everyone, regardless of diagnoses, the premise is that everyone in the world has the personifications of these cognitive processes "living" in their heads. Sometimes these characters are "sleeping" and sometimes they are more "agitated", alluding to when people are more or less activated in relation to cognitive processes. The personification of worry is called Preocupanda and that of rumination, Marrumina. Figure 9.3 depicts the two characters.

The idea is that Preocupanda triggers the siren thoughts when a situation occurs and worries a lot, as opposed to Marrumina who overthinks the situation with rumination and remains inactive in an event. Actually, the idea of personification is to help the patient relate differently to their cognitive processes, making them tell their own bears that they are exaggerating or that a certain event doesn't matter now. This results in a decrease in attentional cognitive syndrome and challenges metacognitive beliefs. The following dialogue illustrates the personification technique with an 8-year-old child.

Therapist: Hello, Alice. How was your week?
Alice: I was very nervous. A lot happened…
Therapist: Do you want to tell me about some of the things that happened?
Alice: I don't know…
Therapist: Alright, let's do this—I'm going to put here on the table some of these cards with emotions, which we've already discussed. We have sadness, fear, anger, disgust. Do any of these have to do with what you felt during this week?
Alice points to sadness and fear.

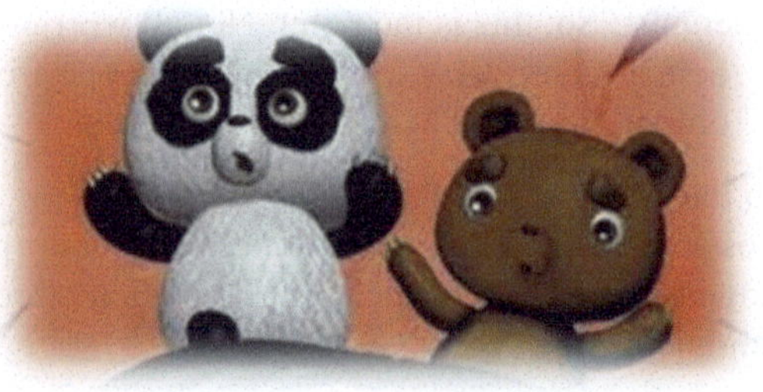

Fig. 9.3 Preocupanda and Marrumina. (Source: Hirata & Gabriel, 2018)

Therapist: Great, thank you for pointing that out to me, Alice. Now let's talk about what made you feel sad or afraid. Do you want to talk?

Alice: My dog, Tobias, got sick. He's in the vet hospital.

Therapist: Oh, I'm very sorry about that and I hope he gets well soon.

Alice: Me too…

Therapist: Maybe we can talk a little more about what you're feeling and how this situation is bothering you. I have here two characters that live in our heads and I think they are working a lot now in yours. Want to meet them?

Alice: Okay…

Therapist: This is Preocupanda, a panda bear that worries. He lives in our heads and keeps triggering siren thoughts like "everything is going to go wrong"; "nobody is going to like you" or "I'm going to fail". He keeps trying to guess all the bad things that can happen. Sometimes he helps us by reminding us of important things, but many times he just makes a lot of noise. Can you identify any siren thoughts from your Preocupanda?

Alice: I think he's saying that Tobias is going to die or that it's going to take a long time to get better.

Therapist: Did the vet say that was going to happen?

Alice: No, he said he's going to get better. But I still think he's going to die.

Therapist: So, it's your Preocupanda saying that. He's triggering a very loud siren and when you keep focusing on that siren, you become more anxious and sadder.

Alice: It's…

Therapist: Let's then talk here with the Worrier. Let's tell him that we know he wants to help, alert, but in fact he is exaggerating. Let's try to just observe him talking, while knowing that it's just chatter.

Alice: Worrier, I know you want to help, but now you are exaggerating.

Therapist: Can you notice the difference, Alice? Between looking at the siren all the time and not stopping to look and being able to realize that it is excessively loud?

Alice: Yes.

Therapist: So, we can practice this throughout the week. Let's separate the sirens that help from those that don't help and, when we realize that some are exaggerated, what are we going to do?

Alice: Tell the Worrier that they are exaggerating.

The dialogue with Alice allows us to observe the use of the character Worrier as a form of detached mindfulness. By realizing that paying too much attention to the Worrier's sirens, she becomes more anxious and sadder, Alice can become aware that it is not always worth stopping to listen to what the character has to say, thus avoiding entering the SCA. In addition, metacognitive beliefs can also be worked on, in the sense that Alice can be asked what she thinks or feels about her own Worrier, as in the passage below.

Therapist: Alice, now that we know the Worrier and have seen how he works, let's talk a little about what you think of him. If you were to choose some of his qualities, which ones would you select? (the therapist can put papers with the qualities written to facilitate the process).

Alice: He is exaggerated, nervous, and useful.
Therapist: Can you explain when he is exaggerated, nervous, and useful?
Alice: When I need to study for a test, he is useful, because he reminds me to study, but when I am taking the test, he is nervous and exaggerated. He says that I won't be able to answer anything.
Therapist: Right. And when he is nervous and exaggerated, what does he do?
Alice: He turns on many sirens and talks non-stop!
Therapist: At those times does it seem like he has no control?
Alice: Yes!

In the dialogue, one can perceive the identification of a positive belief about worry ("worry can be useful") and also a negative one ("worry is uncontrollable"). Thus, in a playful way, it is possible to work with TMC with children or people of other age groups without the use of terms that may be little understandable. For intervention with teenagers or adults, other characters can be used.

Although in the literature there are indications that TMC is more suitable for some specific mental disorders such as OCD (Rees & Koesveld, 2008; Andouz, 2006), GAD (Van der Heiden et al., 2012; Wells & King, 2006), PTSD (Normann & Morina, 2018) and depression (Normann & Morina, 2018), for example, it is important to emphasize that the process of the attention-emotion dyad is universal as well as the processes of worry and rumination.

Conclusion: Metacognitive Therapy as a Transdiagnostic Treatment

Regardless of the presence or absence of diagnoses, both the conceptualization and the techniques of TMC can be applied to a wide range of clinical cases. It is common for patients to complain of "excessive worries" or "excessive guilt", "excessive jealousy" etc. All these complaints can be addressed within a metacognitive perspective. However, instead of the focus of intervention being on the content of these cognitions, it will be on the relationship itself that the individual has with these thoughts, on how he directs attention to these cognitions, and how much he has learned to interpret cognitive processes such as worry and rumination.

References

Andouz, Z. (2006). [Efficacy and effectiveness of Wells's metacognitive model in treating a case of obsessive-compulsive disorder]. *Iranian Journal of Psychiatry and Clinical Psychology, 12*, 59–66.
Beck, A. T. (1976). *Cognitive therapy and the emotional disorders*. Meridian.
Fisher, P., & Wells, A. (2009). *Metacognitive therapy*. Routledge.

Flavell, J. H. (1979). Metacognition and cognitive monitoring: A new area of cognitive developmental inquiry. *American Psychologist, 34*, 906–911.
Hirata, H. P., & Gabriel, S. A. (2017). Utilizando a Terapia Metacognitiva com Crianças. In C. B. Neufeld, E. M. O. Falcone, B. Rangé. (Orgs.). *PROcognitiva: programa de atualização em terapia cognitivo-comportamental*. Ciclo 4, V.3. Porto Alegre: Artmed Panamericana.
Hirata, H. P., & Gabriel, S. A. (2018). *Preocupanda & Marrumina: entendendo a preocupação e a ruminação na criança*. Sinopsys.
Moses, L. J., & Baird, J. A. (2001). Metacognition. In R. A. Wilson; F. F. Keil (Ed). *The MIT encyclopedia of the cognitive sciences* (pp. 533–535). Cambridge: The MIT Press.
Normann, N., & Morina, N. (2018). The efficacy of metacognitve therapy: A systematic review and meta-analysis. *Frontiers in Psychology, 9*, 1–14.
Rees, C. S., & Koesveld, K. E. (2008). An open trial of group metacognitive therapy for obsessive-compulsive disorder. *Journal of Behavior Therapy, 39*, 451–458.
Van der Heiden, C., et al. (2012). Randomized controlled trial on the effectiveness of metacognitive therapy and intolerance-of-uncertainty therapy for generalized anxiety disorder. *Behavior Research and Therapy, 50*, 100–109.
Wells. (2006). Detached mindfulness in cognitive therapy: A metacognitive analysis and techniques. *Journal of Rational-Emotive and Cognitive Behaviour Therapy, 23*, 337–355.
Wells, A. (2009). *Metacognitive therapy for anxiety and depression*. Guilford Press.
Wells, A., & King, P. (2006). Metacognitive therapy for generalized anxiety disorder: An open trial. *Journal of Behavior Therapy and Experimental Psychiatry, 37*, 206–212.
Wells, A., & Matthews, G. (1994). *Attention and emotion: A clinical perspective*. Erlbaum.

Chapter 10
Compassion-Focused Therapy: A Transdiagnostic Approach to Self-Criticism in Clinical Practice

Maria Amélia Penido and Luiz Fellipe Rocha

Historical Aspects

Compassion-focused therapy (CFT) was proposed by British psychologist Paul Gilbert (2009, 2010) with a focus on the transdiagnostic process of self-criticism. Although relatively recent, its origins date back to the 1980s. When applying traditional Cognitive Therapy to depressive patients, Gilbert realized the importance of, not only restructuring the content of dysfunctional cognitions, but also changing the 'emotional tone' of these cognitions (Gilbert, 2022a). In his observations, he concluded that patients with high levels of shame and self-criticism tend to elaborate new perspectives and coping thoughts in a 'mental voice tone' that is cold, intimidating, or aggressive, which blocks the effectiveness of cognitive restructuring. Thus, his efforts began in conceiving an intervention capable of building and strengthening a warm, empathetic, and compassionate stance of patients towards themselves.

In general, Western psychology had, for a long time, a predominantly individualistic focus, pessimistic about human nature, and influenced by a biomedical model aimed at treating diseases, which may justify the late interest in compassion (see Penido & Rocha, 2023 for a review). However, this reality begins to change at the end of the twentieth century and the beginning of the twenty-first century with the incorporation of elements of Eastern psychology—particularly contemplative practices—by Western psychology. Some psychotherapeutic approaches are born from this meeting of cultures, such as Dialectical Behavior Therapy (DBT),

M. A. Penido (✉)
Rio de Janeiro, Brasil

L. F. Rocha
Rio de Janeiro, Brasil
e-mail: luiz.rocha@uerj.br

A. C. Ornelas (ed.), *Transdiagnostic Approaches in Cognitive Behavioral Therapy*, https://doi.org/10.1007/978-3-031-63494-9_10

Mindfulness-Based Cognitive Therapy (MBCT), and Acceptance and Commitment Therapy (ACT).

In this context, Gilbert and Irons (2005) develop an interest in the Buddhist tradition and begin to focus their studies on compassion as a central psychological concept:

> [...] if compassion is a healing process, as Buddhism suggests it is, then we should make this central to our investigations of exactly what it is, and how it works. We need to know how Western science can aid us in understanding the processes involved in compassion and how to cultivate it in our relationships with ourselves, with others, and in our political deliberations. (Gilbert & Irons, 2005, p. 3)

Compassionate Mind Training was developed; a psychological intervention that combines different cognitive-behavioral techniques with the aim of helping people with self-criticism to distance themselves from the internal relationship a dominant-subordinate relationship and to develop a more self-compassionate relationship (Gilbert & Irons, 2005). Therefore, Compassionate Mind Training consists of a series of activities that focus on developing compassionate attributes and skills, aiming at emotional regulation. As can be observed, even though Compassionate Mind Training was based on principles developed by Gilbert since the 1980s, it did not propose a model of psychotherapy.

Compassion-Focused Therapy (CFT) was proposed later in an article entitled 'Introducing Compassion-Focused Therapy', published in 2009, as "an integrated and multimodal approach that draws from evolutionary, social, developmental, and Buddhist psychology, as well as neuroscience" (Gilbert, 2009, p. 199). A more comprehensive text on the approach was published the following year in a book format; 'Compassion Focused Therapy' (Gilbert, 2010), in the series 'CBT Distinctive Features'. Since then, numerous book chapters, books, and scientific articles have been published annually, including a series of meta-analyses that examined the overall efficacy of CFT in positive and negative mental health outcomes (Petrocchi et al., 2023).

Comprehensive Model

CFT can be defined as a process-based therapy whose model is based on a biopsychosocial science informed by evolutionary theory (Gilbert, 2010, 2022a, b). In this sense, it highlights the importance of the interaction and integration of multiple psychological, biological, and social processes in the development of body and mind states. In addition, its philosophical position understands human beings as an emerging species in the flow of life, as part of the evolution of mammals, more specifically, primates.

Its model is built on four basic assumptions (Gilbert, 2010, 2022a, b):

- The human brain is formed by a more primitive part (i.e., 'old brain') and another more recent in evolutionary history (i.e., 'new brain');

- Our emotional states are regulated by at least three main types of neurophysiological systems;
- Compassion is an attitude that can be practiced with the aim of activating the calming system;
- Compassion can flow in three different directions: towards oneself, towards other living beings, and from others to oneself.

The human brain, as a product shaped by millions of years of evolution, developed in a series of stages that progressively added layers to its primitive bases to facilitate survival and reproduction (Gilbert, 2010, 2022a). From this knowledge, CFT assumes the coexistence of two brains. On one side, is the 'old brain', whose structures are also present in the brains of other animals. This brain contains functions (i.e., avoiding harm, seeking resources, and resting and digesting) and basic emotions (e.g., fear, sadness, joy...). On the other side, we have the 'new brain', the part that makes us human, and is linked to the prefrontal cortex endowed with the capacity for complex thinking, reflection, and self-awareness.

These 'two brains' can function and interact in ways that are alien to our will and often conflict, causing problems. This phenomenon is called "complicated brain" in CFT. One of the capabilities of the new brain is to consider the future and predict events that may or may not happen, which tends to trigger the old brain's threat protection capacity, generating anxiety and safety-seeking behaviors. Although this has brought evolutionary advantages, if it happens too frequently or out of context, it can cause psychological suffering and illness. In this sense, it becomes necessary to have a better understanding of how this brain works.

Inspired by the affective neuroscience of evolution, Gilbert (2009, 2010) assumes the existence of three main neurophysiological systems that regulate our emotions and guide our biosocial goals and motivations. These systems are guided by the basic functions of the old brain and are connected to neuro-hormonal circuits. The system focuses on threats and self-protection (or just the threat system) that allows the individual to stay alert and respond quickly to identified threats, motivating the search for safety in response to danger stimuli. This system is linked to the activation of the sympathetic nervous system and the Hypothalamus-Pituitary-Adrenal (HPA) axis, mainly releasing the hormone cortisol. Although the threat system has a primarily adaptive function, many mental health problems are related to it, especially if it is overdeveloped, sensitive, biased, or confused.

In general, the threat system is more related to psychopathology due to the processes involved in its activation, such as neuro-hormonal mechanisms (for example, cortisol response), negative emotions or emotional states (for example, stress, fear, anxiety, and anger), biased cognitive processing (for example, hypervigilance and worry), and often dysfunctional safety strategies (for example, avoidance and self-criticism). The drive system—also called the stimulus, incentive, and resource-seeking systems—functions to motivate the search for resources and rewards, guiding the development of desires and goals. This system provokes positive emotional states, such as excitement and pleasure, that energize attention, advancement, and resource seeking (e.g., food, status, and sexual opportunities). This happens mainly through the release of dopamine.

The drive and threat systems interact in such a way that the search for resources may be connected to the attempt to fight against threats or avoid them, projecting a safety-seeking strategy for negative events (for example, pursuing high standards to avoid feelings of inferiority). At the same time, the hindrance of the action system (for example, when goals are not achieved) tends to provoke the activation of the threat system, generating a negative emotional response.

The soothing system, in turn, helps balance the other two systems through the activation of the parasympathetic nervous system and the release of oxytocin, being a source of security, well-being, tranquility, and contentment. That is, it is a source of positive affect different from those aroused by the drive system (i.e., excitement, enthusiasm…). It produces a state of contentment with how things are, without seeking or desiring resources or rewards. It is also different from the simple absence of threats, which can generate boredom or a sense of lack. This system was shaped by evolution to be activated by attachment behaviors (for example, nourishment, validation, empathy, and compassion), as it brought benefits to the species, such as the survival of offspring and the development of useful alliances.

In view of this, CFT calls on the capabilities of the 'new brain' to understand and transform the functioning of these three emotional regulation systems when they are causing problems and psychological suffering for the patient. It is assumed that the soothing system is underdeveloped for self-critical individuals (Boersma et al., 2015).

Indeed, evidence suggests that a lack of self-compassion is linked to insecure attachment and childhood maltreatment and may mediate the effect of insecure attachment on emotional dysregulation. In addition, evidence shows that, in self-critical individuals, high levels of negative affect are accompanied by low levels of positive affect (Gilbert et al., 2008).

The goal of CFT is to balance the three systems, taking into account the context of each client. The focus is not on just increasing the soothing system since compassionate motivation operates in all three systems. For example, in the case of a client who is trapped in an abusive relationship, the most compassionate attitude will be to activate their threat system to leave the relationship (Cattani et al., 2020).

In CFT, compassion is defined as a sensitive attitude towards suffering (one's own and that of others), accompanied by a commitment to alleviate or prevent it (Gilbert, 2010, 2022b). Two psychologies or two mental states of compassion can be observed in this definition.

The first psychology of compassion involves coming into contact with suffering, rather than avoiding or distancing oneself from it. For this, some attributes are necessary (Irons & Beaumont, 2018):

- Caring for well-being: genuine interest in how the person feels
- Sensitivity: being sensitive/open to one's own (and others') feelings, emotions, thoughts, and behaviors
- Sympathy: motivation to 'care'. Being available to be emotionally moved by pain and suffering

- Tolerance of discomfort: being able to manage one's own discomfort arising from the connection with suffering
- Empathy: the ability to put oneself in the place of another, as if one were the other, without, however, losing the condition of 'as if'
- Non-judgment: involves an acceptance of the difficult things that one's complex mind can bring to the world and our relationships, trying not to judge, criticize, or condemn

The second psychology of compassion consists of engaging in behaviors for the relief and prevention of suffering. For this, some skills are essential (Irons & Beaumont, 2018):

- Compassionate attention: the ability to come into contact with pain without over-identifying with it; noticing other elements involved to generate a balanced perspective
- Compassionate imagination: the ability to use the 'new brain' to bring to mind useful compassionate memories, images, and/or a sense of identity
- Compassionate thinking and reasoning: the ability to use our rational minds, looking at the evidence and bringing a balanced perspective
- Compassionate behavior: the ability to wisely work on actions and behaviors that help us alleviate our own distress and suffering, or that of another person
- Compassionate sensory focus: the ability to have a sensory focus, stimulating our different senses (for example, smell, hearing, touch), to help stimulate affiliative positive emotion and, more broadly, the conditions for compassion
- Compassionate feelings: the ability to invest time generating and practicing certain positive emotions linked to compassion, such as warmth, kindness, friendship, and contentment

Compassion, as proposed by CFT, can flow in three distinct directions (Irons & Beaumont, 2018). When we direct compassion towards others, we are sensitive to their suffering and mobilized to help them. This attitude generates positive outcomes in the one who experiences it through the activation of the soothing system. It also tends to have a reassuring effect on the one who is receiving compassion. It requires, however, being open to receiving care, affection, and support from others.

Finally, one can direct compassion towards their own suffering through a self-compassionate stance. However, it is not always easy to give and receive compassion. What has been observed over the years of research and practice in CFT, is that there may be blocks or resistances to compassion and affiliative connections. This phenomenon, called fear of compassion, can involve negative beliefs about (self)compassion and/or conditioning mechanisms, when the desire for closeness is associated with aversive stimuli or punishment (Gilbert, 2010).

Transdiagnostic Process: Self-Criticism

CFT was developed to work primarily with patients with high levels of self-criticism, a process understood as "an inner sense of disconnection through our own hostility towards (parts of) ourselves" (Gilbert, 2022c, p. 164). It is not, therefore, about interventions in the sense of diminishing constructive self-criticism or the desire for self-improvement.

The focus is on self-criticism that activates the threat system, generating a physiological stress response. Self-criticism is related to negative outcomes in mental health, such as depressive and anxious symptoms, and low adherence to psychotherapy (Gilbert, 2010, 2022c). In addition, self-criticism has also been pointed out as a transdiagnostic process (Gilbert & Irons, 2005), as it plays an important role in the etiology, maintenance, and course of various psychopathological states, such as eating disorders (Williams & Levinson, 2022). Gilbert distinguishes three functions of self-criticism (1) the inadequate self, where self-criticism has the function of correcting and avoiding mistakes or motivating the client to improve; (2) the hated self, where this process has the function of pursuing, hurting, and destroying the person (present in more severe mental disorders and quite resistant to change); and (3) the inhibited self, whose function is to silence and humble the client, preventing arrogance, growth, and self-assertion (Gilbert, 2022c). From the functional analysis of self-criticism, CFT proposes to understand it in terms of safety-seeking strategies (Gilbert, 2010, 2020; Gilbert & Irons, 2005).

Self-criticism can be used in order to protect oneself from one's most central fears. A person may, for example, believe that their self-criticism protects them from being a total failure. Other people may fear becoming arrogant, aggressive, unpleasant, relaxed, lazy, or out of control if they let go of their self-criticism. CFT seeks to replace self-criticism with other more functional strategies for dealing with threats, mainly, from the development of the compassionate self. The compassionate self does not fight the critical self in an aggressive or combative way, but sympathizes with the fears behind it and sets boundaries in an assertive way (Gilbert, 2022c).

Therapeutic Work

The therapeutic efficacy of CFT in working with shame and self-criticism in the context of a variety of clinical disorders and non-clinical populations is becoming increasingly well established (Kirby, 2017; Leaviss & Uttley, 2015; Matos et al., 2017). In a recent systematic review and meta-analysis (Millard et al., 2023) on the effects of CFT in clinical populations, improvements were found in both clinical symptoms, such as depressive and eating disorder symptoms, and in compassion-based outcomes, such as self-compassion, self-criticism, fear of self-compassion, and self-reassurance compared to control groups.

Alternatively, studies point to Compassion Focused Therapy (CFT) and self-compassion as effective for the care of excessive self-criticism (Leaviss & Uttley, 2015). Developing compassion is a factor that appears associated with a decrease in the feeling of exclusion and a decrease in self-criticism and shame.

Clinical work with self-criticism seeks to find ways to change the internal dialogue of threat to compassionate ways of treating oneself (Gilbert, 2009). The therapeutic process in CFT presents concepts and techniques that are integrated from psychoeducation, case formulation, and therapeutic relationship, resulting in an individualized treatment plan that focuses on compassionate mind training. Compassionate mind training seeks to build the skills to develop and strengthen a version of the self that incorporates compassion (Gilbert, 2022d).

In general, we can highlight some fundamental aspects of the therapeutic process in CFT, such as: 1. Therapeutic relationship: the therapist acts as a model for the development of the compassionate mind, in addition to acting as a base and safe harbor, this posture of the therapist contributes to the "de-shaming" procedure, that is, de-shaming (Gilbert, 2022b).

The relationship of acceptance promotes an environment in which the patient can explore their problems, understanding the external and internal influences that contributed to their problems, removing the shame of being the sole cause of their own difficulties, and moving them towards a posture of responsibility to alleviate and prevent their own suffering (Gilbert, 2022e). 2. Psychoeducation: a fundamental aspect of CFT, the patient learns about the complicated brain and its consequences, also about the three emotional regulation systems, compassion, and flows of compassion. This information helps eliminate some misconceptions about compassion, which then allows clients to be open to perceive how it can help them, reducing fears and blocks of compassion (Gilbert, 2022d).

When psychoeducating clients about compassion in CFT, it is crucial to distinguish compassion from concepts such as kindness or gentleness, as they can reinforce a mistaken stereotype that being compassionate is akin to being a docile person, who accepts aggressions or does not feel anger (Cattani et al., 2020). 3. Case formulation: the process of organizing patient information and problems according to CFT concepts usually helps patients feel less shame about their current difficulties.

The formulation seeks to understand the historical, genetic, and social influences that contributed to the client developing the defense strategies and problems that led them to therapy (Gilbert, 2022e). 4. Compassionate Mind Training (CMT): seeks to help people access and stimulate their affiliative motivations, emotions, and competencies, which can be part of the experience of the compassionate self. This includes interventions such as the use of breathing, posture, facial expressions, voice tones, and other exercises. It seeks to develop in therapeutic work a series of compassion cultivation exercises through attentional training and mindfulness practice, cultivation of compassionate self-identity, use of compassionate mental images, compassionate writing, and the act of regularly performing compassionate behaviors. These interventions are planned to stimulate the motivation, emotion, and cognition systems that corroborate compassion, so that they can become more integrated into the sense of self-identity.

In CMT, clients are introduced to the CFT viewpoint that the mind is made up of several different versions of the self, what is called multiple self or multiple mind. The client learns to identify and dialogue with their internal parts, such as the anxious self, the angry self, the sad self, and the compassionate self. The goal is to normalize the existence of conflicting and complex internal perspectives, which, for clients with a lot of self-criticism and shame about their internal world, is a relief, as they often feel that their emotional "confusion" is a sign that they are psychologically "broken".

Then, the compassionate self is brought to the fore to mentalize and empathize with the other states of the self and to guide the client in making the decision to deal with the problem that evoked the anxious, angry, and sad self (Cattani et al., 2020). The goal of compassionate mind training through different techniques is to develop compassionate reasoning, allowing the development of a healthy relationship with an integrated self, while balancing the client's emotional regulation and always taking into account the life context of each individual.

Description of a Clinical Case in CFT

JS, woman, heterosexual, 43 years old, single, dentist, white, middle class, living in the northeast, has a 4-year-old son. JS defines herself as a very worried and anxious person, she has had episodes of depression throughout her life, but currently the complaint is about symptoms of anxiety, exaggerated self-criticism, and chronic worry. She reports that she has always been worried and anxious since childhood and attributes these characteristics to her childhood, especially the relationship with her mother. She describes her mother as a very difficult and controlling person, she never felt loved by her. She describes her mother as extremely critical of her, nothing she did was ever good enough, her mother was very verbally aggressive, calling her a stupid idiot very often, in addition to reporting that she suffered physical punishments daily, whenever she did something that her mother did not like she was beaten, she remembers with much pain from childhood. She had a good relationship with her father, but he worked a lot and did not get involved in her relationship with her mother and generally defended the mother as authority asking the daughter to accept and try to improve the behavior and relationship. She is the oldest of three children and reports that the mother was different with the brothers; she never hit or spoke ill of them. She understands that this happened because the brothers were men. In her childhood the figure she remembers with affection, by whom she felt loved was a housemaid who helped take care of her, she always had a lot of affection for this caregiver and considered her as family. She died 2 years ago, and it was a very difficult loss. The relationship with her father was good, she felt loved and he always supported her financially, but she never understood the reason he did not protect her from her mother, she considered him negligent in relation to this aspect.

The father died 4 years ago and it was also a very difficult loss. She does not have a good relationship with her brothers and does not speak to her mother. She believes that the family rejects her and therefore prefers not to live with them. She has a little support network, and few friends. She does not consider herself a very sociable person, she thinks that generally people do not like her. She always had a lot of performance anxiety, especially with tests, she had difficulty finishing college because of this anxiety and considers herself a stupid person, slow who takes longer than others to learn. During college, she had difficult depression and was medicated and underwent therapy. She improved and did not open a depression case again, but anxiety is constant in her life. She went to college in another city far from the family and after graduating lived outside of the country, but when her father became ill she returned to the same city as the family and lives there until today. She has never been married, had some boyfriends, but considers that the relationships were toxic, as they were abusive people and she never felt loved. She had her daughter through artificial insemination as an independent parent and considers it the best thing she did in her life. She is very fulfilled as a mother. The current complaint of chronic worry, exaggerated self-criticism, and anxiety was aggravated by a financial difficulty after the father's death. She works as a dental radiologist diagnosing exams from home and depends on contracts with city clinics. Her income depends on how many exams she can diagnose and this generates a lot of worry. In addition to worrying about being able to handle the diagnoses, she tends to be very demanding with her performance, does not consider herself good at what she does and therefore reports that she is hard on herself with her performance and checks the diagnosis many times, looking to do it perfectly, which takes time, and hinders her productivity. She has a lot of anxiety with work and constantly has self-critical thoughts like: "I'm not good", "I'm not doing my best" "I should try harder" "I need to study more" "I need to balance work and my daughter otherwise I'm not a good mother" "they will realize that my diagnoses are not good and will no longer send me exams" "I'm going to run out of money" "I'm going to fail in my life" "I don't do anything 'right'" "I'm very tired and stupid" "I can't study or learn" "I'm going to fail and I'll never be loved by anyone". This pattern of self-criticism and worry results in a lot of difficulty concentrating, anxiety attacks, difficulty sleeping, and chronic fatigue. She presents physical symptoms such as recurring migraines, body pain, and daytime sleepiness. At the moment she is not taking any medication and thinks that taking medicine means she is not capable of handling life on her own. In addition to concerns about work and financial life, she also criticizes her body a lot and reports eating excessively due to anxiety, considers herself ugly and overweight, can't lose weight and has a lot of difficulty doing physical activity, she is always very tired. She has little leisure time, what she likes most is to be with her daughter, but as she has difficulty handling work, she ends up having to work on weekends to deliver all the reports and this prevents her from paying attention to her daughter. She tends to blame and criticize herself for this. She has had therapy before, she considers that it helped her with depression but not with anxiety. Her goal is to better handle anxiety to be able to handle life.

Treatment Plan

Establish the therapeutic relationship: the therapist in CFT functions as a model of the compassionate mind, does not adopt a posture that emphasizes techniques or problem solving but validation and acceptance. Highly self-critical patients may have safety behaviors activated in the relationship with the therapist, especially at the beginning of the relationship. Safety behaviors were conceptualized as self-protection strategies employed to mitigate fears of exposing negative attributes in social situations (Moscovitch, 2009). Just as self-critical patients fear exposing perceived flaws and being the target of criticism, they also simultaneously fear expressions of compassion and affection (Cunha et al., 2015).

One of the characteristics that can hinder the construction of an affective relationship with the patient is the fear of receiving compassion. This fear has been associated with early experiences of shame, and individuals who experience greater fears of compassion recall fewer positive and affiliative memories from childhood (Matos et al., 2017; Silva et al., 2019). In the case of JS, her childhood was very difficult and she suffered a traumatic and dysfunctional relationship with an aggressive mother. It is believed that these experiences form the basis for maladaptive social schemas that make it difficult for anxious individuals to feel safe in their social environments (Kelly & Dupasquier, 2016), leading them to interpret compassion as threatening.

The fear of receiving compassion can center specifically around feelings related to devaluation, the belief that the need to receive compassion from others is a sign of weakness, or that compassion is equivalent to pity (Gilbert et al., 2011). For fear of rejection or criticism, these patients may resist manifestations of affection, empathy, and compassion from the therapist. The therapist needs to consider that the patient's thoughts may not only focus on fears of evaluation, but that even the supportive responses of others can be perceived as threatening.

The therapist can then investigate whether these fears are present, assess how the patient deals with receiving help, demonstrate positive affection, receive affection, feel self-compassion. Psychoeducating the patient about these skills and the fear of compassion can contribute to the therapeutic relationship. The fact that the person sought therapy can be used as a starting point to question beliefs that warmth and kindness are threatening. Using behavioral experiments to test whether receiving compassion is really threatening, assessing whether receiving such compassion from others and from the therapist is as bad as they expected can help clients acquire useful experimental evidence. Behavioral experiments in which the clients themselves offer compassion to others, or asking clients to reflect on their own previous experiences of giving compassion can help them recognize that care can be driven by connection and empathy, rather than pity for the person in danger. Learning to accept the compassion of others as genuine and well-intentioned can reduce perceptions of threat, encouraging them to reveal their authentic selves to develop deeper and more meaningful experiences, starting with the relationship with the therapist (Ho et al., 2021).

During this first phase of TFC, the clinician used reflective listening to help JS feel heard, understood, accepted, validated, and valued. In addition, reflective listening aided in guided discovery, for the discovery of her own intrinsic wisdom, a key aspect of TFC.

Case Formulation in CFT

The case formulation in TFC aims to collaboratively build an understanding of the current problem and maintenance factors and serves as a guide for treatment. In addition, it helps the client to have a clear understanding of their problem, and to practice an attitude of validation about their functioning when they realize that it is not their fault, thus the feeling of self-recrimination and shame are worked on in the formulation. For this, it is important to explore historical influences, such as childhood memories, especially memories related to acceptance and safety, as well as memories linked to fears and threats.

In JS's case, the memories were linked to a bad relationship with her mother and not feeling accepted, validated, and loved. She developed an inadequate sense of self and always felt pressured to perform well. The memories linked to a sense of worth were from the affection received by the caregiver whom she considered her foster mother. For her, others were judgmental and self-focused, rarely available, and critical.

After accessing historical influences and significant childhood experiences, the therapist and client seek to identify the main fears that derived from these experiences. In her case, fear of failure, and fear of being judged and unloved greatly impact her. The fear of being negatively evaluated by others, of failing in life, and not being able to handle everything became constant concerns in her life.

The main internal fears were about being a fraud and failing, losing control and discovering that she would not be worthy of love. The key fears, internal and external, are very painful, and people try in some way to alleviate and avoid this pain by creating defense and avoidance strategies. Perfectionism in reviewing work, working hard and always striving to the maximum, constant self-criticism to try to socially adapt and produce, overeating, constantly worrying about the future are examples of strategies adopted by JS. She constantly feels insecure and strives for perfection, never being able to value previous successes, adopting a posture of self-attack and criticism in relation to the self. Worry and self-criticism are seen by her as strategies that protect her from her own feelings of inadequacy and shame, functioning as motivators toward success and perfection and consequent social acceptance. Unfortunately, these strategies that seem to help, in fact reinforce the problem. As a consequence of these strategies, JS ends up isolating herself from people, avoiding social contact, spends a lot of time working, and misses opportunities to build social support. JS feels alone, unloved, tired, and stressed. Sharing the formulation helped to provide a rationale for treatment, tasks and goals were discussed and established with JS. In this case, the goals of JS's treatment were to work with her main fears, explore changes in her safety behaviors, reconnect with people, and manage anxiety, chronic worry, self-criticism and compensation in food.

The adoption of a compassion-focused approach was proposed, as a kind of "antidote" to worry, self-demand and self-criticism, and JS agreed to proceed in this way. Secondly, having a clear formulation of her case helped her to de-shame and not blame herself for the situation she was in. She was able to see how the version of herself that she became was shaped by her experiences. De-shaming and accepting her responsibility, but not blame, were themes that continued to open. The entire treatment plan, starting with the formulation, has been described.

Psychoeducation in CFT and its evolutionary basis: at this stage the client is psychoeducated about the complicated brain, the three emotional regulation systems, and then the concept of compassion, self-compassion, fears, and resistances of compassion are introduced through texts, films, breathing exercises and *mindfulness*. The purpose of this phase of the treatment plan was to help JS develop awareness and understanding about the mind, especially understanding the evolutionary nature of the brain, the adaptive functions of the brain that helped human survival and reproduction, but that also come with various trade-offs, resulting in greater suffering. In CFT, this is colloquially called "our complicated brain". JS was very aware of the threat system from the fight/flight/freeze perspective and its relationship with self-criticism, shame, and worry, and she strongly identified with the drive system, especially the need for attainment and achievement. At one point in the session, she said: "I think what I do is use the drive system to compensate for the threat system." This self-discovery of her "threat-based drive" was very important for her ongoing understanding of herself and how her worries are maintained. JS was less familiar with the soothing system, which refers to the important role of affiliation, connection, care, nurturing, and sense of social safety in human survival. When discussing the soothing system, JS began to cry. After a few moments, she said: "This is the part that always lacked." She went on to reflect on how she never felt nurtured as a child. She found it very difficult to relate to the idea of self-compassion. The hypersocial nature of humans and the way humans monitor themselves in relation to others, including how we ourselves can be seen in the minds of others was discussed. She could see how fearful imagination, worry about the future, and ruminative recall of the past, were the drivers of her self-criticism. She also said: "I'm always so worried about what other people think. Sometimes I feel like I lose myself in my worries about others, trying to please them or be approved." At this point, the therapist introduced self-criticism as part of the discussion and the way this arises from complicated loops in the brain, like old brain anxiety and disgust mixing with the new brain and its fearful imagination and worries that others see her as inadequate or unworthy. Thus, JS and the therapist came to an agreement about her "complicated brain" and the role of worry, rumination, and self-criticism in her problems. At this stage of treatment, the concept of compassion was introduced in detail from psychoeducation. Compassion was explored further by inviting JS to describe her own experiences of receiving compassion. She found this difficult at first, however, she persisted and remembered her caregiver, who always treated her with compassion. JS described the caregiver as having a series of qualities:

warmth and care, wisdom and good sense, acceptance and non-judgment, fun and humor. The idea of compassionate eating was introduced at this stage of therapy.

Compassionate mind training: Introduction of image exercises for compassion included: safe place, ideal compassionate figure, and learning to practice the compassionate mind in therapy and at home from guided practices of compassionate meditation. Six compassionate skills were worked on: imagination, reasoning, behavior, physical sensation, emotion, and attention. Exploring the multiple selves from the anxious self, angry self, sad self, and compassionate self. Working with client's values and motivation from the values the development of the compassionate self-connected to values. Psychoeducation about self-criticism, exploring difficult memories and managing with self-compassion. Compassion pause, writing compassionate letters to the different selves. Use of image exercises and empty chair in the process, developing the compassionate mind and compassion skills. The therapist conducted an analysis of the function of her "anxious self" through an exercise of imagination. In this exercise, JS was invited to bring to mind a situation that triggers anxiety. She was asked to choose something of moderate severity to start with. She chose the reports she can't make. When discussing what she thought could be the function of the anxious self, she said: "Well, it motivates me, makes me work harder and do better." JS and the therapist then explored her greatest fears linked to this situation. She said: "I would probably fall apart, do nothing, achieve nothing and, therefore, everyone's opinions about me would be correct. I can't handle life". JS and the therapist continued with the exercise, which involved closing her eyes and bringing to mind her anxious self, as if it could take on its own form, and imagine what it might look like and sound like, what it might say and how it might be feeling about her. The effect of this imagination exercise for JS left her feeling empty, frustrated, sad, and unmotivated. She then activated the compassionate self, and repeated the same exercise in relation to the problem with the reports, but this time remembering the compassionate self, as if it could take on its own form, and imagine what it might look like and sound like, what the compassionate self might say, how it felt about her and, most importantly, what kind of relationship the compassionate self would like to have with her. JS was invited to consider what message the compassionate self would like to convey to the anxious self? How can the compassionate self-validate the pain and suffering of the anxious self? How can the compassionate self-reassure the anxious self? What encouragement can the compassionate self-offer? The treatment plan continued to strengthen the compassionate self in different situations and contexts of her life. Therefore, CFT contributed to cultivating compassion, promoting affect regulation, and managing worry, anxiety and self-criticism, which was especially beneficial for her case.

Conclusion

Clinical research in CBT has recently sought to understand how the process of change in psychotherapy occurs. The question is no longer which global intervention works for whom, or which techniques work for which disorder, but rather to understand which basic processes are involved in the change achieved in psychotherapy. The goal is to discover which basic biopsychosocial process can be accessed and modified in a specific patient, with a specific goal in a certain situation and then understand the components that need to be modified for healthy functioning (Hayes & Hofmann, 2018). Self-criticism is considered a transdiagnostic psychological process associated with worse mental health that has been empirically investigated. Appearing to be associated with different psychopathologies, consequent forms of clinical intervention that contribute to reducing self-criticism have also been investigated. The development of greater self-compassion contributes to reducing self-criticism, with self-compassion being a predictor of mental health, thus clinical interventions that focus on developing self-compassion have emerged as an alternative for self-critical patients.

Clinical psychology should be increasingly based on an integrative, evolutionary, and contextual biopsychosocial science, focusing on understanding the process of change in psychotherapy. For Gilbert (2019), future therapies will also focus more on the moral aspects of therapy and will address the need to promote pro-social and ethical behaviors with oneself and others.

References

Boersma, K., Håkanson, A., Salomonsson, E., et al. (2015). Compassion focused therapy to counteract shame, self-criticism and isolation. A replicated single case experimental study for individuals with social anxiety. *Journal of Contemporary Psychotherapy, 45*, 89–98. https://doi.org/10.1007/s10879-014-9286-8

Cattani, K., Griner, D., Erekson, D., Burlingame, G., Beecher, M., & Alldredge, C. (2020). *Compassion focused group therapy for college counseling centers*. Routledge Mental Health.

Cunha, M., Pereira, C., Galhardo, A., Couto, M., & Massano-Cardoso, I. (2015). Social anxiety in adolescents: The role of early negative memories and fear of compassion. *European Psychiatry, 30*(S1), 1–1. https://doi.org/10.1016/S0924-9338(15)30336-9

Gilbert, P. (2009). Introducing compassion-focused therapy. *Advances in Psychiatric Treatment, 15*(3), 199–208. https://doi.org/10.1192/apt.bp.107.005264

Gilbert, P. (2010). *Compassion focused therapy: Distinctive features*. Routledge.

Gilbert, P. (2019). Psychotherapy for the 21st century: An integrative, evolutionary, contextual, biopsychosocial approach. *Psychology and Psychotherapy: Theory, Research and Practice, 92*(2), 164–189. https://doi.org/10.1111/papt.12226

Gilbert, P. (2022a). Setting the scene: Psychotherapy at a crossroads and a compassionate way forward. In P. Gilbert & G. Simos (Eds.), *Compassion focused therapy: Clinical practice and applications* (pp. 3–23). Routledge.

Gilbert, P. (2022b). Compassion focused therapy: An evolution-informed, biopsychosocial approach to psychotherapy: History and challenge. In P. Gilbert & G. Simos (Eds.), *Compassion focused therapy: Clinical practice and applications* (pp. 24–89). Routledge.

Gilbert, P. (2022c). Internal shame and self-disconnection: From hostile self-criticism to compassionate self-correction and guidance. In P. Gilbert & G. Simos (Eds.), *Compassion focused therapy: Clinical practice and applications* (pp. 164–206). Routledge.

Gilbert, P. (2022d). Compassionate mind training: Key themes. In P. Gilbert & G. Simos (Eds.), *Compassion focused therapy: Clinical practice and applications* (pp. 273–312). Routledge.

Gilbert, P. (2022e). Formulation and fears, blocks, and resistances. In P. Gilbert & G. Simos (Eds.), *Compassion focused therapy: Clinical practice and applications* (pp. 207–239). Routledge.

Gilbert, P., & Irons, C. (2005). Focused therapies and compassionate mind training for and self-attacking. In P. Gilbert (Ed.), *Compassion: Conceptualisations, research and use in psychotherapy* (pp. 263–325). Routledge.

Gilbert, P., McEwan, K., Mitra, R., Franks, L., Richeter, A., & Rockliff, H. (2008). Feeling safe and content: A specific affect regulation system? Relationship to depression, anxiety, stress, and self-criticism. *The Journal of Positive Psychology*, 182–191. https://doi.org/10.1080/17439760801999461

Gilbert, P., McEwan, K., Matos, M., & Rivis, A. (2011). Fears of compassion: Development of three self-report measures. *Psychology and Psychotherapy: Theory, Research and Practice, 84*(3), 239–255. https://doi.org/10.1348/147608310X526511

Gilbert, P. (2020). Compassion: From its evolution to a psychotherapy. *Frontiers in Psychology, 11*, 586161. https://doi.org/10.3389/fpsyg.2020.586161. PMID: 33362650; PMCID: PMC7762265.

Hayes, S. C., & Hofmann, S. G. (Eds.). (2018). *Process-based CBT: The science and core clinical competencies of cognitive behavioral therapy*. New Harbinger. [Links].

Ho, J. T. K., Dupasquier, R. J., Scarfe, M. L., & Moscovitch, D. A. (2021). Fears of receiving compassion from others predict safety behaviour use in social anxiety disorder over and above fears of negative self-portrayal. *Journal of Anxiety Disorders, 80*, 102387, ISSN 0887-6185. https://doi.org/10.1016/j.janxdis.2021.102387

Irons, Dr. C., & Beaumont, E. (2018). *The compassionate mind workbook: A step-by-step guide to developing your compassionate self*. Robinson.

Kelly, A. C., & Dupasquier, J. (2016). Social safeness mediates the relationship between recalled parental warmth and the capacity for self-compassion and receiving compassion. *Personality and Individual Differences, 89*, 157–161. https://doi.org/10.1016/j.paid.2015.10.017

Kirby, J. N. (2017). Compassion interventions: The programmes, the evidence, and implications for research and practice. *Psychology and Psychotherapy: Theory, Research and Practice, 90*, 432–455. https://doi.org/10.1111/papt.12104

Leaviss, J., & Uttley, L. (2015). Psychotherapeutic benefits of compassion-focused therapy: An early systematic review. *Psychological Medicine, 45*(5), 927–945. https://doi.org/10.1017/S0033291714002141

Matos, M., Duarte, J., & Pinto-Gouveia, J. (2017). The origins of fears of compassion: Shame and lack of safeness memories, fears of compassion and psychopathology. *The Journal of Psychology Interdisciplinary and Applied, 151*(8), 804–819. https://doi.org/10.1080/00223980.2017.1393380

Millard, L. A., Wan, M. W., Smith, D. M., & Wittkowski, A. (2023). The effectiveness of compassion focused therapy with clinical populations: A systematic review and meta-analysis. *Journal of Affective Disorders, 326*, 168–192. https://doi.org/10.1016/j.jad.2023.01.010

Moscovitch, D. A. (2009). What is the core fear in social phobia? A new model to facilitate individualized case conceptualization and treatment. *Cognitive and Behavioral Practice, 16*(2), 123–134. https://doi.org/10.1016/j.cbpra.2008.04.002

Penido, M. A., & Rocha, L. F. D. d. (2023). Compaixão e psicoterapias: desafios e evidências científicas. In C. B. Neufeld, E. M. d. O. Falcone, & B. Rangé (Eds.), *Procognitiva Programa de atualização em terapia cognitivo-comportamental: ciclo 10* (pp. 9–46). Artmed Panamericana.

Petrocchi, N., Ottaviani, C., Cheli, S., Matos, M., Baldi, B., Basran, J. K., & Gilbert, P. (2023). The impact of compassion-focused therapy on positive and negative mental health outcomes:

Results of a series of meta-analyses. *Clinical Psychology: Science and Practice*. https://doi.org/10.1037/cps0000193

Silva, C., Ferreira, C., Mendes, A. L., & Marta-Simões, J. (2019). The relation of early positive emotional memories to women's social safeness: The role of shame and fear of receiving compassion. *Women & Health, 59*(4), 420–432. https://doi.org/10.1080/03630242.2018.1487906

Williams, B. M., & Levinson, C. A. (2022). A model of self-criticism as a transdiagnostic mechanism of eating disorder comorbidity: A review. *New Ideas in Psychology, 66*, 100949. https://doi.org/10.1016/j.newideapsych.2022.100949

Chapter 11
The Unified Protocol Approach for Emotional Disorders

Ana Claudia Ornelas and Marcio Moreira da Silva

Introduction

The unified protocol was created to cover various emotional disorders, through a refinement of techniques that promote changes and strengthen the skills to cope with stressful situations. The main advantage of the unified protocol is to develop a treatment common to different specific disorders and their comorbidities (Barlow et al., 2011; Button et al., 2012; DeOrnelas Maia et al., 2013; Sauer-Zavala et al., 2017). The same authors endorse that the previous alternative would be the use of several specific protocols for each treatment. Other research is being conducted and establishes data on the protocols for both specific treatments for anxiety or depression and for treatments of emotional disorders in general, the transdiagnostics, and these validate this freedom in choosing the best intervention regarding the conceptualization of the clinical case (Donker et al., 2009; Marcal, 2005; Schweizer et al., 2020). The intervention with the unified protocol is as efficient as the interventions used with the specific protocols, but more economical and faster for individuals who present heterogeneous psychological disorders or different diagnoses (Steele et al., 2018; Schweizer et al., 2020). Thus, transdiagnostic treatments offer a promising path when it comes to emotional disorders with comorbidities, as well as complex presentations regularly seen in clinical practice. This chapter aims to describe the steps of the unified protocol and present examples of the techniques used during the 8 modules, with a clinical case.

A. C. Ornelas (✉)
Sunshine Therapy, Malden, MA, USA

M. M. da Silva
CEMED, Missao Velha, Brazil

A. C. Ornelas (ed.), *Transdiagnostic Approaches in Cognitive Behavioral Therapy*, https://doi.org/10.1007/978-3-031-63494-9_11

The Steps of the Unified Protocol

Initially, the client undergoes an initial evaluation that will allow the therapist to carry out the clinical conceptualization. At this stage it is up to the therapist to use the anamnesis interview as an initial step, in addition to evaluating mood and anxiety with the use of a validated or reliable inventory or questionnaire for such formulation. DeOrnelas Maia et al. (2013, 2015) in their studies point out that during the initial evaluation process, the therapist can teach the client to understand what psychotherapy is and what the model of the CBT approach is. From there, the therapist will investigate and certify with the client about the pros and cons of being in therapy. The therapist and client will talk thoroughly about the plans and strategies of treatment with the use of the unified protocol. Then, the client and therapist work together to define the goals that will be formulated from the conceptualization of the case. By placing the objectives and goals in the treatment plan, the client and therapist can stipulate how long they would like to carry out the unified protocol and the number of sessions, regarding the frequency and duration of them. At this step, strategies for problem solving are planned. In the unified protocol, despite having a plan regarding the number of sessions, both the clinical conceptualization and the treatment time can be reviewed, if the therapist and the client have this need. Table 11.1 represents the eight steps of the unified protocol, containing the number of sessions for each module.

Table 11.1 The UP's modules, number of sessions and objectives

Modules	Sessions	Objectives
1. Increased motivation and commitment to therapy	1–2	Motivation for the therapy proposal
2. Help the client identify, recognize, and evaluate emotional responses	1–2	Through psychoeducation, the therapist guides the client about the emotional components common in emotional disorders
3. Assess emotional awareness and focus on the present moment	1–2	Promote awareness and acceptance of one's emotions
4. Perception and cognitive assessment	1–2	Teach the client to practice cognitive flexibility, through strategies for identifying and restructuring dysfunctional beliefs
5. Assessment of emotional avoidance—emotions and intentions drive behaviors and thoughts	1–2	Observe the standards of avoidance behaviors
6. Behaviors and tolerance to physical sensations	1–2	Clients are motivated to perceive physical symptoms through hyperventilation techniques
7. Exposure	4–8	Through a position of emotions, apply gradual exposure from the lowest intensity to the greater, understanding the mechanism of adaptation
8. Relapse prevention	1–2	Review of treatment and application of the same under the same or different conditions

Barlow et al. (2011) introduced some general models of questions that the therapist can use to activate the client's motivation for therapy. The questions are open-ended and serve to reflect on the advantages and disadvantages of undergoing the therapeutic process.

- When you think about change, do you make choices based on any previous evidence that has worked? Give an example from your experience.
- When you avoid a situation or a relationship with someone, does it increase your confidence? Give an example from your experience.
- Have your goals and objectives been achieved according to the strategies and timeline you set? Give an example from your experience.
- Have you recently experienced thoughts, sensations, and attitudes that motivate new life plans and increase your self-confidence? Give an example from your experience.

Process of Restructuring Core Beliefs

From the decision to start treatment, the client will learn to recognize and differentiate thoughts, emotions, and behaviors. In addition to observing, according to the model of rational emotive and behavioral therapy (REBT), the antecedents, responses, and consequences that label irrational beliefs about the individual's view of themselves, others, and the world will be noticed (Cape et al., 2010; Craddock & Owen, 2010).

The therapist discusses with the client examples and their own social models from their daily routine. At this step, the therapist can offer a task using a chart to facilitate the client's monitoring of their beliefs and events that occur in their routine during the week. By realizing that the antecedent factors are the situations, and the moment when they occurred, the responses included thoughts, emotions, and behaviors obtained in the experienced situation, and the consequences are the learnings that validate a new skill or cognitive construction, the client begins to have a better interaction with their own experience and is reinforced in their self-knowledge. Barlow et al. (2011) present in their studies a proposal of REBT which demonstrates the antecedent processes, the responses, and the consequences with the defeats of beliefs and the emergence of new patterns generating a new experience throughout the individual's life.

Process of Emotion Regulation

For the individual to evaluate and reevaluate what they are thinking, feeling, and how they will act in response to thoughts and sensations, they need, however, to learn to identify which emotion and thoughts about this emotion are associated.

From this model, the unified protocol will help the client understand emotional functions as a learning process and strengthening of new understandings and behaviors about emotions. Emotions direct new thoughts and actions (Barlow et al., 2011; Sauer-Zavala et al., 2017; Steele et al., 2018).

Mindfulness

For several years now, *mindfulness* (full attention) has been a recurring concept in our daily lives. The explanation of this concept is very simple, but not always easy to practice, and it is transversal to all routine (and non-routine) activities of our life. Full attention is a practice that consists of directing all attention to the present moment (Aldao & Nolen-Hoeksema, 2010). Thus, it becomes possible to focus only on the experience that is being lived, allowing thoughts to flow naturally without judgments. This practice is defined as the awareness that arises when attention is paid to the present moment.

The mental state of being "*mindful*" is characterized by the self-regulation of attention to the present experience, in an open, curious, broad, and tolerant attitude, directed at all phenomena that manifest in the mind consciously, that is, all types of thoughts, fantasies, memories, sensations, and emotions perceived in the field of attention are perceived and accepted as they are. While in the Buddhist context it carries the meaning of keeping in mind the correct information (Ruggero et al., 2019).

Training can be carried out daily through learning that usually takes place through guided meditation techniques and other related exercises, such as stretching, yoga, Pilates, or even simple breathing, allowing the individual a broad awareness of their mental processes and actions.

Interoceptive Exposure

Interoceptive exposure aims to correct the catastrophic interpretations of the physical symptoms felt by patients as part of anticipatory anxiety or a panic attack. With interoceptive exposure, patients undergo gradual exposure to feel comfortable with the sensations (Barlow et al., 2011; DeOrnelas Maia et al., 2015; Ruggero et al., 2019). This exposure is done through the intentional provocation of symptoms using physical exercises. There is a list of exercises that can be used for the therapist to teach the client to confront physical sensations.

It can be, for example, with continued physical activation, or even breathing only through the mouth until hyperventilation is provoked, spinning in the swivel chair several times, or any effort that is continued for 1–3 min. The physical sensations are similar to an anxiety crisis, the mouth becomes dry, sensations of heat, tachycardia, tremors, dizziness, or even panting. The role of the therapist in this procedure is to teach the client to stabilize with breathing techniques and mindfulness (Barlow et al., 2011; Johnston et al., 2011; Lambert, 2013; Powers et al., 2006).

In addition to direct training to feel comfortable with these sensations (where patients learn to experience sensations as strange or uncomfortable, rather than scary), interoceptive exposure also allows patients to identify automatic thoughts and catastrophic interpretations associated with physical sensations and correct them (Barlow et al., 2011; Johnston et al., 2011; Lambert, 2013; Powers et al., 2006).

The exercises of interoceptive exposure can function as a preparation for in vivo exposure. Interoceptive exposure interventions are typically introduced in the session and completed at least twice by the therapist and patient together, focusing on helping patients do nothing to try to control or minimize sensations. Home practice of the exercises is then indicated, with the aim that the patient becomes accustomed to the sensations by the next weekly session.

Finally, patients are asked to complete the interoceptive exposure in sessions where they are afraid of panic, so that comfort with the sensations can be learned in that context. This practice of interoceptive exposure outside the session provides a useful smooth transition to in vivo exposure (Barlow et al., 2011; Johnston et al., 2011; Lambert, 2013; Powers et al., 2006). In vivo exposure is the main intervention applied to overcome agoraphobic avoidance. To plan in vivo exposure, the patient must make a list of places or situations that they have avoided due to fears, and also record the level of anxiety and automatic thoughts that arise in these situations. This list should be arranged in a hierarchy according to the level of difficulty in facing places and situations. In vivo exposure exercises are initiated by situations considered less anxiety-provoking and that the patient is willing to face. To be effective, exposure must be prolonged in time (stay in a given situation for approximately twice the time it takes to feel comfortable in that situation), repeated frequently, and the level of anxiety must be felt during the task and monitored by both the patient and the therapist (Barlow et al., 2011; Johnston et al., 2011; Lambert, 2013; Powers et al., 2006).

Clinical Case

For example, a case of a 40-year-old client who is unemployed, with a wife and 2 children aged 4 and 6 years, identifies that he is tense, has constant nausea, poor concentration, frustration, rapid and short breathing, tachycardia (physical symptoms of anxiety); observes his thoughts allied to the physical symptoms which are: "I only have enough to pay the bills and support my family for 30 days, and what if I take too long to find a new job?"; "No one will want to hire me if they notice that I am distressed and without concentration"; "I am weak and without an exit"; and has compulsive eating behaviors, spends money on scratch-off lottery tickets, and avoids going to look for a new job.

For this case, the steps of the unified protocol were fundamental and the techniques used under the light of CBT:

1. The therapist can use the pros and cons to motivate this client to look for other possibilities according his thoughts. For example, for this client's concerned: "I only have enough to pay the bills and support my family for 30 days, and what if I take too long to find a new job?" The therapist reentered with the client that if it happens, he can find a solution if it occurs. But at this moment, he has 30 days to look for a new job to pay his bills. Whether or not he finds a new job, he is still dealing with worries, lack of concentration, weakness, and gets his bills paid. So, try to be in the present moment and make an action plan.
2. The therapist will also use psychoeducation about anxiety symptoms and cognitive distortion "I am weak and without an exit", for example: Have you been in that position before? What did you think would happen? Those questions can be cultivated by guided discovery with Socratic questioning, the arrow descent, advantages and disadvantages, and the motivational interview. Those interventions include open-ended questions to the client, such as: What could you do if the worst scenario occurs? And have you thought if it can be different? What are some other actions you could take? Have you thought about the advantages to changing your food habits? The therapeutic objective is finding the core beliefs about those automatic thoughts.
3. The therapist will use Mindfulness techniques with this client to achieve awareness and self-regulation of emotions in the present moment; interoceptive breathing, exposure, and relapse prevention. They can plan a hierarchy list and make an action plan to face each situation that can change the pattern or drive the emotion to manage it.

During treatment with the unified protocol, the client will develop resources and skills to achieve some goals:

1. Evaluate and reassess their cognitive and emotional flexibility through the activations of the process in therapy. The steps to be reviewed in the unified protocol are, for example, understanding and regulating emotions, and accepting and committing to perceive them as a natural part of life. The techniques used to achieve these goals are: mindfulness, exposure, and psychoeducation.
2. Sensations (emotional and physiological) direct thoughts (cognitions) and behaviors (actions). The techniques that activate sensations and provide decision-making are: exposure, guided discovery, mindfulness.
3. Antecedent events provoke responses and the consequences of these become new learning; if positive for the client it becomes reinforcing of a new behavior. Rational Emotive and Behavioral Therapy (REBT) promotes this step in the process of CBT intervention.
4. The skills learned can strengthen a new desired model of action/attitude of the client. Self-confidence and well-being increase the evidence of a new behavior model and functional pattern. The techniques that enable this improvement are: Psychoeducation, REBT approach, techniques such as guided discovery, interoceptive breathing, exposure, and mindfulness.
5. The client learns to be aware of the situation and the present moment, beginning to recognize that emotions are part of life and what matters most is to be an

observer in managing them with kindness and curiosity, suspending their own judgments. The technique of mindfulness enables achieving this view of compassion, kindness, and curiosity in the face of situations and interpretations experienced by the individual.

6. The client will learn cognitive flexibility and begin to use it in the process of emotion regulation. The techniques of psychoeducation, and the use of REBT, mindfulness. and guided discovery promote this cognitive flexibility to the individual.
7. Emotions direct behaviors, this shows that the client becomes active in the management and use of strategies for balance and self-confidence. The client and the therapist in this step are validated with the skills learned during each session.
8. The client will use as a safety method the prevention of anticipated emotions, that is, they will observe and manage the occurrence of situations that are happening in reality and will not validate those imagined. The unified protocol promotes a new meaning for the individual's life, where new resources are learned to manage and regulate emotions.

Conclusion

When psychotherapists begin their learning in CBT, they can sometimes make the mistake of seeing this approach as just a set of techniques or interventions. In this way, they forget the main therapeutic resources for the treatment result to be a predictor of a favorable prognosis for both the client and the psychologist: clinical conceptualization and the development of a collaborative therapeutic relationship. With this, they go through some of the most important aspects of CBT too quickly, and go directly to perform the intervention with the techniques, such as, guided discovery or even exposure, mentioned in the course of this chapter.

It is very easy to fall into this trap since CBT is known for its effective interventions and the fact that patients usually engage well in specific exercises. By performing clinical conceptualization, the therapist has the possibility to improve both a therapeutic alliance and plan treatment under the individual condition that is brought by the client, who becomes active in their process of change. This process is called a collaborative therapeutic relationship.

The transdiagnostic view allows the mental health professional a non-stigmatized and non-formatted look at generalized conduct. In addition, transdiagnostic approaches tend to overcome therapy management for people with unspecific problems of criteria that close mental health diagnoses. Third-generation CBT offers an evidence-based transdiagnostic intervention and serves a range of typical diagnoses of the general population that may be associated with anxiety and/or secondary depression.

The development of a unified protocol based on CBT has been bringing promising results that promote a more human and individualized therapeutic relationship and provides the client with improvements in their emotional, cognitive and social functioning. Without the pretension of becoming a different protocol from others, but with important contributions from an approach that already has considerable acceptance by the population and also by mental health professionals.

References

Aldao, A., & Nolen-Hoeksema, S. (2010). Specificity of cognitive emotion regulation strategies: A transdiagnostic examination. *Behaviour Research and Therapy, 48*(10), 974–983.

Barlow, D. H., Farchione, T. J., Firholme, C. P., Ellard, K. K., Boisseau, C. L., Allen, L. B., & Ehrenreich- May, J. (2011). *Unified protocol for transdiagnostic treatment of emociotional disorders*. Therapist Guide. ThatWork. Oxford University Press.

Button, K. S., Wiles, N. J., Lewis, G., Peters, T. J., & Kessler, D. (2012). Factors associated with differential response to online cognitive behavioural therapy. *Social Psychiatry and Psychiatric Epidemiology, 47*(5), 827–833.

Cape, J., Whittington, C., Buszewicz, M., Wallace, P., & Underwood, L. (2010). Brief psychological therapies for anxiety and depression in primary care: Meta-analysis and meta-regression. *BMC Medicine, 25*, 8–38.

Craddock, N., & Owen, M. J. (2010). The Kraepelinian dichotomy—Going, going...but still not gone. *The British Journal of Psychiatry, 196*, 92–95.

DeOrnelas Maia, A. C., et al. (2013). Transdiagnostic treatment using a unified protocol: Application for patients with a range of comorbid mood and anxiety disorders. *Trends in Psychiatry and Psychotherapy*. [online], *35*(2), 134–140.

DeOrnelas Maia, A. C., Nardi, A. E., & Cardoso, A. (2015). The utilization of unified protocols in behavioral cognitive therapy in transdiagnostic group subjects: A clinical trial. *Journal of Affective Disorders, 172*, 179–183.

Donker, T., Griffiths, K. M., Cuijpers, P., & Christensen, H. (2009). Psychoeducation for depression, anxiety and psychological distress: A meta-analysis. *BMC Medicine, 16*, 7–79.

Johnston, L., Titov, N., Andrews, G., Spence, J., & Dear, B. F. (2011). A RCT of a transdiagnostic internet-delivered treatment for three anxiety disorders: Examination of support roles and disorder-specific outcomes. *PLoS One, 6*(11), e28079.

Lambert, M. J. (2013). Outcome in psychotherapy: The past and important advances. *Psychotherapy (Chicago, Ill.), 50*(1), 42–51.

Marçal, J. V. (2005). Estabelecendo Objetivos na Prática Clínica: Quais Caminhos Seguir? Revista Brasileira de Terapia Comportamental e Cognitiva.Vol. VII, nº 2, 231-245. Recuperado em 03 de dezembro de 2023, de http://pepsic.bvsalud.org/scielo.php?script=sci_arttext&pid=S1517-55452005000200008&lng=pt&tlng=pt

Powers, M. B., Smits, J. A. J., Leyro, T. M., & Otto, M. W. (2006). Translational research perspectives on maximizing the effectiveness of exposure therapy. In D. C. S. Richard & D. L. Lauterbach (Eds.), *Comprehensive handbook of exposure therapies* (pp. 106–160). Academic.

Ruggero, C. J., Kotov, R., Hopwood, C. J., First, M., Clark, L. A., Skodol, A. E., et al. (2019). Integrating the Hierarchical Taxon-omy of Psychopathology (HiTOP) into clinical practice. *Journal of Consulting and Clinical Psychology, 87*, 1069–1084.

Sauer-Zavala, S., Gutner, C. A., Farchione, T. J., Boettcher, H. T., Bullis, J. R., & Barlow, D. H. (2017). Current definitions of "transdiagnostic" in treatment development: A search for consensus. *Behavior Therapy, 48*, 128–138.

Schweizer, T. H., Snyder, H. R., Young, J. F., & Hankin, B. L. (2020). The breadth and potency of transdiagnostic cognitive risks for psycho-pathology in youth. *Journal of Consulting and Clinical Psychology, 88*, 196–211.

Steele, S. J., Farchione, T. J., Cassiello-Robbins, C., Ametaj, A., Sbi, S., Sauer-Zavala, S., & Barlow, D. H. (2018). Efficacy of the Unified Protocol for transdiagnostic treatment of comorbid psychopathology accompanying emotional disorders compared to treatments targeting single disorders. *Journal of Psychiatric Research, 104*, 211–216.

Chapter 12
Stress and Burnout: Current Cognitive Behavioral Therapy Interventions from the Perspective of Transdiagnostic Approaches

Juliana Caversan de Barros and Lucia Emmanoel Novaes Malagris

Introduction

Stress and burnout are phenomena that demand a lot of attention from psychotherapists, as they can bring great harm to an individual's quality of life. It is essential that the professional knows what stress is and what burnout syndrome (BS) is, as well as the relationship between the two, which is one of the first steps for effective interventions to be implemented. Considering that these phenomena can be present in a variety of clinical complaints, a cognitive-behavioral approach based on the transdiagnostic model proves to be a good treatment option for diagnostic cases that include stress and BS.

A Cognitive-Behavioral Therapy (CBT) approach aimed at patients with various criteria needs to be based on common processes to a wide range of individual complaints that appear in the clinical context. The transdiagnostic model (de Ornelas, 2020) brings together proven evidence-based approaches and effective strategies to meet these demands, develop psychological flexibility, promote behavioral changes and restore the quality of life of affected individuals.

This chapter aims to discuss a treatment alternative based on CBT according to the transdiagnostic model, specifically, from the perspective of Process-Based Therapy (PBT) (Hofmann et al., 2023), which is one of the therapies based on the transdiagnostic model. The treatment cores available to manage stress and BS present in other clinical complaints, such as those focusing on attention, cognition, affect, motivation, and explicit behavior, will be addressed.

J. C. de Barros (✉)
Niterói, RJ, Brazil

L. E. N. Malagris
Rio de Janeiro, RJ, Brazil

A. C. Ornelas (ed.), *Transdiagnostic Approaches in Cognitive Behavioral Therapy*, https://doi.org/10.1007/978-3-031-63494-9_12

First, the topics of stress and BS will be explained, followed by the interaction between these phenomena and other clinical conditions. PBT will be addressed and its applicability will be illustrated in a clinical case.

Stress

Stress is present in everyone's daily life, but often it is not properly understood. Therefore, it can be neglected in its capacity to, when excessive or poorly managed, bring great harm to quality of life. However, it is important to note that stress is necessary for survival, only becoming a problem when it goes beyond the individual's resources and when there are no appropriate strategies for its management.

Stress constitutes a break in the body's homeostasis in the face of a threat or challenge. The phenomenon was initially named by Hans Selye as the Syndrome of Being Just Sick because he observed a group of symptoms that repeated in some individuals and, later, as General Adaptation Syndrome (GAS), since he concluded that it referred to a series of symptoms aimed at adjusting the body in response to a certain stimulus (Selye, 1965). Later he named it stress, using the word used in engineering, making an analogy with what happens to a bridge when subjected to an overload beyond its capacity (Selye, 1976).

Selye (1976) developed his studies leading to the triphasic model of stress which consisted of three phases: alert, resistance, and exhaustion. Lipp, after many years of studies and clinical experience in the field of stress, developed the quadriphasic model, understanding that the process occurs in four phases: alert, resistance, near-exhaustion, and exhaustion (Lipp, 2000; Lipp & Malagris, 2011). The alert phase is the first and occurs when the body encounters a stressor that requires a confrontation, causing a break in homeostasis and a readiness to deal with the situation. Often the individual confronts the stressor and returns to its natural homeostasis.

The resistance phase comes next, when the organism has reached its limit for confrontation and needs recovery to return to its adaptation. The near-exhaustion phase, according to Lipp (2000), occurs when the organism cannot recover in the second phase, possibly because the stressor remains present (in a real or imaginary way) or because the individual did not have appropriate strategies to seek recovery. In near-exhaustion, as the name suggests, the organism is being defeated in the fight for balance, but always fighting. If it does not recover, it evolves to the fourth phase, exhaustion. This phase constitutes an excessive wear of the organism in the struggle to deal with the stressor and for rebalancing, but, due to the presence of the stressor(s), the individual's vulnerabilities and/or lack of adequate tools (strategies), there was no success. It is important to remember that the stress process is always a search for adaptation/homeostasis, even in advanced stages. That is, the organism undergoes physiological changes in an attempt to balance itself (Chu et al., 2021). It does not always succeed and can reach advanced stages and develop diseases, physical and emotional, which will also become sources of stress for the person who already suffers, bringing more suffering and risk to health.

The symptoms of stress vary according to the phase and knowing them favors the diagnosis of the level of stress in which the individual is and, thus, an appropriate therapeutic approach can be implemented. For example, in the alert phase, which is considered positive stress, it is common for the person to become more hyperactive, may have insomnia, have peaks of blood pressure, tachycardia, among other symptoms that are related to the necessary activation to face a stressful situation. In the resistance and near-exhaustion phases, the symptoms are similar, but in the third phase the commitment is greater. In these two phases, it is common to have memory problems, general malaise, constant fatigue, a lot of emotional sensitivity, difficulty concentrating, for example. In the exhaustion phase, which is the most serious phase, people who reach this phase usually feel insomnia, nausea, dizziness, high blood pressure, prolonged skin problems, depression, anxiety, anguish, among others. All symptoms, in their different phases, have physiological correlates responsible for the way the individual manifests stress (Lipp & Malagris, 2011; Straub, 2014; Malagris & Dias, 2019; Chu et al., 2021). The organism, in the fight or flight process, characteristic of stress, uses physiological changes to deal with the stressor and return to its homeostasis.

As Tavares et al. (2000, p. 65) emphasize, "...there is a complex interaction between systems, cells and neurotransmitters, which provide, according to the basal state and the alternative pathways of each organism, responses and behaviors manifestly particular". Stressors can relate to various situations and are dependent on the interpretation that the individual gives to them (Xu et al., 2020). They can come from various areas and contexts, including anticipated threats, against which there is no evidence of occurrence (Malagris & Dias, 2019). That is, the sources of stress can be external or internal. Among the external ones, we can mention losses, unemployment and interpersonal conflicts, among the internal ones we can consider personality traits, behavioral patterns and anxiety. Even if the stressors are related to a specific area, in general, all other areas are compromised (Lipp & Malagris, 2011). It is essential that the individual develops coping strategies in the face of stressors, so as not to reach the exhaustion phase and its serious consequences.

Burnout

When the stressors are present in the occupational area and the individual reaches the exhaustion phase, the Burnout Syndrome (SB) can occur, as Benevides-Pereira (2008) states. As Areosa and Queirós (2020) states that negative work-related interferences on physical and mental health are a public health issue. The World Health Organization (WHO), in 2017, focused on mental health in the workplace for World Health Day. In 2019, burnout was considered an occupational phenomenon in the new International Classification of Diseases—ICD-11 (WHO, 2019). Despite these resolutions being quite recent, research on burnout began in the 1970s by Freudenberger (1974), with the concept being further developed by Maslach and Jackson (1981) who emphasized physical and psychosocial aspects.

Mesquita and Malagris (2020) note that the definition of burnout developed by Maslach and Jackson in 1986 is the most influential today. The authors define it as "a reaction to chronic emotional stress generated through direct and excessive contact with other human beings, present in the routine of health professionals" (Mesquita & Malagris, 2020, p. 66).

According to Maslach and Jackson (1986), burnout involves three dimensions: emotional exhaustion, depersonalization, and low job satisfaction. To diagnose burnout, all three dimensions must be present at high levels. Emotional exhaustion relates to emotional wear and tear due to job demands. Depersonalization, also called cynicism, refers to negative attitudes and feelings directed at people with whom the individual interacts in the workplace, as if it were a dehumanization in serving others. Low job satisfaction reflects the professional's dissatisfaction in their work environment. Some relationships between the dimensions of burnout have been studied. Taris et al. (2005) found in their studies an association between these dimensions, concluding that high levels of exhaustion are associated with high levels of depersonalization over time and that higher levels of depersonalization contributed to higher levels of emotional exhaustion and lower levels of personal accomplishment.

To consider that a person is indeed experiencing burnout, according to Maslach and Jackson (1986), it is necessary for all three dimensions to be present concurrently at a high level. Initially, studies in the field considered that burnout would specifically affect professionals who care for people, however, it has been observed that it can develop in all types of professions (de Aquino et al., 2023). For Areosa and Queirós (2020), burnout refers to one of the pathologies related to overload generated by organizations such as: "high degrees of stress and anxiety; weak levels of autonomy and excessive control over workers; insufficient rewards and lack of recognition; overwork and high emotional demands; deregulation of work collectives and absence of equity; and toxic relationships between workers (degradation of values), likely to increase conflicts" (p. 72). However, it is important to consider the individual with their personal, behavioral, cognitive, and emotional characteristics, which can also contribute along with environmental issues to the development of burnout.

For Maresca et al. (2022), systematic and dysfunctional habits and individual psychological reactions harm personal well-being and constitute burnout generators. The same situation can be faced differently by different people. Some studies focus on coping strategies and have found significant correlations between emotional exhaustion, depersonalization, and dysfunctional coping (Ding et al., 2015, cited by Maresca et al., 2022).

Lazarus and Folkman (1987) classified coping modes based on problems and based on emotion, considering that those based on emotion are harmful to health. It should be emphasized that the damages associated with stress and burnout to the individual's quality of life are many, which requires special attention from health professionals, organizations, the scientific community, and public institutions. Various studies have been presenting intervention proposals.

Interaction Between Stress, Burnout, and Various Diagnoses

Stress and burnout (SB) can be present in a variety of clinical issues and it is essential that the professional knows each of the phenomena in their peculiarities to understand the interaction between them. From this understanding, a transdiagnostic intervention will be possible that contemplates the psychological processes that overlap in the clinical demands treated.

One of the cases where the interaction between stress and another clinical complaint is clearly perceived is social anxiety. According to Goodman et al. (2023), people who suffer from this disorder exhibit maladaptive social and regulatory behaviors that can generate stress. According to the authors, not only the difficulty in social relations in these people is associated with stress, but also other life domains, such as financial difficulties (Fehm et al., 2008, cited by Goodman et al., 2023) and occupational impairment (Moitra et al., 2011, cited by Goodman et al., 2023).

Studies have investigated the relationship of SB with depression, anxiety, and even personality disorders, seeking an understanding that goes beyond organizational variables. Such studies expand the knowledge of this syndrome that brings so much damage to the individual's quality of life. In the specific case of depression, the first scholar on SB already referred to the fact that when a person suffers from the syndrome, they seem depressed and act as such (Freudenberger, 1974).

However, Fischer et al. (2020) concluded in a study with Intensive Care Unit doctors that burnout and depression are related, but are empirically different. These authors emphasize that emotional exhaustion and depersonalization form the core of SB and that it is important to consider the distinctions included in the syndrome for proper diagnosis and treatment. That is, it is observed, according to the studies, that SB involves depression, but it is a phenomenon with its own characteristics despite some similarities. Such similarities, in the logic of the transdiagnostic model, involve maladaptive processes that when managed bring gains for the treatment of both phenomena.

As for the relationship between SB and anxiety, as Guerra (2022) states, these phenomena differ, as SB results from the accumulation of occupational stressors, while anxiety refers to future threats. A literature review conducted by Koutsimani et al. (2019) concluded that anxiety and burnout are different constructs and that there is no overlap between the phenomena, but emphasizes the relationship between them. According to the authors, studies indicate that burnout is a risk factor for anxiety and they cite Koutsimani et al. (2019) who argue that people predisposed to anxiety are also predisposed to SB. Still regarding anxiety, Queirós et al. (2019) conducted a study with nurses and concluded that trait anxiety is a vulnerability factor for burnout, without disregarding organizational aspects. The authors suggest that anxiety management work could contribute to the prevention of SB.

Golonka et al. (2019) also emphasize this connection, especially with the aspect of exhaustion of the syndrome. In their research with workers, Golonka et al. (2019) concluded overlaps of SB both with depression and with anxiety and emphasized the role of the individual and their characteristics in addition to work-related determinants.

Considering that SB has been related to individual issues and not only to the environment, aspects of personality, such as pathological perfectionism, rumination, pessimism, neuroticism, and negative affectivity (Alarcon et al., 2009), should be investigated. It is interesting to study the relationship with personality disorders, such as borderline personality disorder (BPD). Its characteristics such as hypersensitivity to rejection, impulsivity, and affective instability can contribute to problems in the area. Occupational. Studies indicate that people with BPD often have problems in the workplace, such as commitment issues and tumultuous occupational experiences (Skodol et al., 2002).

Bianchi et al. (2018) studied the relationship specifically of BPD in education professionals, based on the observation that people with this disorder often have frequent job changes, go through periods of disability, and tend to be unemployed (Skodol et al., 2002). Bianchi et al. (2018) concluded that there is an association of BPD with SB, suggesting, however, that the problems in the occupational area of these individuals are not related only to a general tendency towards negative emotionality. An overlap of SB with depressive symptoms mediating the relationship between BPD and certain common occupational aspects of these individuals, such as a tendency to unemployment, turnover, and work disability, was observed. It was found that in women there was an association with affective insecurity and impulsivity, characteristics of BPD. In men, an association between SB and affective insecurity was also found, but not with impulsivity. Another interesting finding is that participants with high BPD scores reported more burnout symptoms.

Transdiagnostic Model

The transdiagnostic approach was developed as an alternative to traditional treatment, which often segments and treats disorders based on their specific characteristics. The central idea of the transdiagnostic model is that several psychological disorders have common roots, such as dysfunctional cognitive processes (for example, recurring negative thoughts), emotional difficulties (such as difficulty in regulating emotions), and maladaptive behavioral patterns (such as avoiding feared situations). In the past, a diagnosis with several comorbidities would require the application of multiple treatment protocols and varied therapeutic approaches (de Ornelas, 2020).

Treatments based on the DSM (Diagnostic and Statistical Manual of Mental Disorders) proved to be relatively simplistic models that seemed not to encompass the entirety of the context and experience of patients. Contextual theories came to fill these gaps (Hayes et al., 2023a). Instead of directing treatment to a specific diagnosis, transdiagnostic therapies seek to treat these underlying processes shared by different disorders. Eustis et al. (2020) emphasize that its applicability to a wide range of problems can simplify treatment and make it more efficient and sustainable. In addition, this approach allows treatment to be more flexible and personalized, addressing the patient's problems more broadly, rather than sticking to specific symptoms.

Considering Mansell et al. (2008) understanding that the similarity between disorders is greater than the difference between them, models focused on psychological processes present in various difficulties tend to benefit a much more significant number of demands. The transdiagnostic intervention seeks to treat various psychological disorders through common processes among them, instead of addressing each disorder in isolation. In other words, the focus is not on the specificity of a particular diagnosis, but on identifying and treating underlying psychological patterns and processes that are shared by different disorders.

For Barlow et al. (2020), the perspective of treating comorbid disorders through new unified therapeutic protocols takes into account the application of innovative approaches in the treatment of psychological disorders that coexist in the same individual. Instead of treating each condition separately, the idea is to develop unified approaches that can be effective for multiple disorders. Thus, the transdiagnostic model suggests an approach promising and modern for the treatment of complex psychological conditions, seeking the creation of integrated and unified therapeutic protocols that meet the specific needs of each individual. This reflects an evolution in the understanding and treatment of mental health issues, aiming for a more comprehensive and effective approach (Gallagher et al., 2013).

The treatment with Unified Protocol (UP) in Cognitive-Behavioral Therapy (CBT) developed by David Barlow in 2011 brings this new focus, emphasizing emotional regulation, and as a basic structure the clinical conceptualization with the purpose of identifying the intervening variables that contribute to the problem or diagnostic complaint, the understanding of the dysfunction or function of the problem, and the elaboration of a treatment plan (Barlow, 2016). The aim is for the individual to recognize the intensity, frequency, and persistence of their emotions, aiming to manage them in a way that guides learning and emotional functionality. It is worth noting that the CBT-based UP is just one example of transdiagnostic treatment and that there are other approaches developed and explored in the field of Psychology.

The UP starts from the premise that deficits in the ability to manage emotions, such as avoidance, struggle, and overcompensation, contribute to the triggering and maintenance of emotional disorders. By developing emotional skills strategies, it promotes a broad understanding of what thoughts, feelings, and behaviors are; manages and improves these initially identified emotional and behavioral characteristics, and generates a modification in the functioning of the emotional direction that governs consequential behaviors and thoughts. As a result, it contributes to the improvement of patients' physical and emotional tolerances, to the acquisition of cognitive flexibility and emotional regulation (de Ornelas, 2020).

Process-Based Therapy

Various types of therapeutic interventions have been developed based on the transdiagnostic model, focusing on psychological processes underlying a range of emotional difficulties, among them, Process-Based Therapy (PBT) stands out as a comprehensive and innovative proposal. Being PBT a contemporary approach of CBT, it stands out for directing its focus predominantly to evidence-based processes, connected to procedures backed by proven data, instead of rigidly adhering to protocols intended for the treatment of specific syndromes (Hayes & Hofmann, 2017). This more flexible and personalized perspective seeks to integrate information from various sources and generations of CBT, allowing for more effective adaptation to the individual needs of patients.

Historically, the first therapeutic approaches focused on syndromes and syndromic groups, limiting their ability to encompass all the comorbidities and heterogeneities presented by clients. According to Hofmann and Hayes (2018), the pronounced bias of biomedicalization, with excessive emphasis on protocols for specific syndromes, resulted in the neglect of various crucial aspects for clinical issues. This led to a failure to adequately meet individual needs and, consequently, the numerous specificities associated with them. This approach also reduced the emphasis on the quality of the changes generated by the treatment.

With the evolution to the third Generation of Cognitive-Behavioral Therapy (CBT), there was an increase in the emphasis on change processes, which are responsible for driving positive transformations during treatment (Hofmann & Hayes, 2019). By addressing and working these underlying mechanisms, therapy aims to facilitate the achievement of desired goals. Third-generation CBT approaches highlight the importance of understanding and directing the dynamic processes that lead to significant changes, making treatment more effective and adapted to individual needs.

Recent studies, conducted post-DSM-based treatments, indicate that by incorporating comprehensive and evidence-based data from all generations of CBT, professionals in the field have the opportunity to offer more effective assistance to their patients. According to Hofmann et al. (2023) argue that integrating information from the various generations of CBT allows for a more complete and adaptable understanding of individual needs, contributing to more personalized and efficient therapeutic approaches in the treatment of mental disorders. This movement reflects an evolution in clinical practice, leveraging knowledge accumulated over time to benefit mental care.

Adopting the understanding of the therapeutic process as inherently non-linear, characterized by complexity and dynamism, forming an intricate network of multiple interactive processes, where emotional, cognitive, behavioral, and environmental factors are constantly intertwined (Hayes et al., 2023a), TBP emerges with the role of promoting the transformation of inadequate patterns to more appropriate ones, seeking not only change but also sustainable maintenance. This approach does not represent a completely new treatment method, but rather an innovative approach in the conception of therapeutic methods. It is based on the functional analysis of behavior, which includes the individual (idiographic) assessment of the target behavior and the context in which it occurs. Its goal is to clarify the functional relationship of the variables that contribute to the manifestation of behavior (Hayes et al., 2019).

TBP presents the elaboration of a metamodel of sets of adaptive and maladaptive change processes, with six psychological dimensions and two additional levels of analysis crossed with the four main evolutionary questions, widely applicable, transdiagnostic, and versatile (Hofmann et al., 2023). It covers four main evolutionary concepts to understand the dynamics of psychological processes: variation, selection, retention, and context. From Charles Darwin's perspective of highlighting contextual interference in human behavior, Hofmann et al. (2023) emphasize that Psychology can develop interventions that take this understanding into account to enhance therapeutic gains. Understanding the context as key to psychological processes helps to expand the possibilities of therapeutic interventions for clinical challenges.

The intervention structure of TBP explained by Hofmann et al. (2023) can be understood according to the following evolutionary concepts:—The concept of variation refers to the diversity of psychological processes that individuals can manifest in response to various challenges and situations. As a context changes, variation is necessary. It is essential to have flexibility to find ways to adjust to a constantly changing environment. When there is no variation, one can fail to adjust to the context. To vary means to make choices that work in that context. TBP explores the range of responses and strategies that a client uses in different contexts.—Regarding selection, this encompasses the process by which certain psychological processes are preferentially chosen or reinforced based on their perceived effectiveness in facing challenges. Some choices lead to more successful outcomes than others.

From this understanding, it is possible to understand how the client's psychological processes were selected over time in response to specific situations. This may involve identifying patterns of thought, emotions, or behaviors that have been repeatedly reinforced or chosen. In relation to retention, it includes the persistence or maintenance over time of the psychological processes that have been selected. From this perspective, the therapist can explore why certain psychological processes persist, even though they may be maladaptive. This may include identifying intrinsic or extrinsic rewards associated with these processes. According to TBP, adaptation is achieved by presenting healthy variation, with selection and retention to a given context. On the other hand, psychopathology is understood as specific context problems of these aspects, which can occur at various dimensions and levels (Hayes et al., 2023a).

Regarding the six dimensions, cognition is considered (how the individual interprets life events), affect (emotional reactions to life circumstances), attention (the focus direction given by each person in their internal and external experiences), self (self-image and self-perception), motivation (the magnitude of change possibilities), and explicit behavior (how the individual acts in situations). In all these dimensions, adaptive and maladaptive aspects can be presented (Hofmann et al., 2023).

By integrating these concepts, PBT equips therapists to help their clients understand how their psychological processes have developed in response to their life experiences. The process-based approach allows for the identification of dysfunctional patterns that can be targets for therapeutic intervention. It also facilitates engagement towards change, helping clients develop and reinforce more adaptive psychological processes in response to current challenges.

Application of Process-Based Therapy for a Transdiagnostic Case of Social Anxiety, Stress, and Burnout

The work environment can contain numerous stress sources as it involves interpersonal interactions, hierarchy relations, goals, and deadlines to be met, among others. When such external sources combine with individual internal stressors, a magnification of their impact on the individual's organism is observed, making them more vulnerable to developing a high level of stress and, consequently, more predisposed to developing burnout. Individuals with social anxiety disorder, for example, tend to perceive social events as more threatening than they actually are, experiencing deregulated emotions and engaging in avoidance and escape behavior from feared situations. Such behaviors provide short-term relief but increase insecurity in the face of long-term personal interactions, causing these individuals to engage in an unproductive functioning circle. As they become increasingly vulnerable to socialization, they suffer intense wear and tear that can increasingly compromise their survival in the work environment.

Considering the complex interaction of variables between stress and social anxiety disorder, it is possible to consider that the presence of high social insecurity in the work environment can predispose the individual to stress and, consequently to burnout, just as a burnout condition can predispose to the triggering of social insecurity components (Goodman et al., 2023).

According to Aderka and Hofmann (2023), an approach like PBT, which integrates strategies for the psychological processes present in transdiagnostic cases, is promising for effective and sustainable behavioral change. The construction of the process-based treatment model for a transdiagnostic case of social anxiety, stress, and burnout will be presented below.

Clinical Case and Application of PBT

Pedro, 42 years old, sought therapy due to a high level of stress, with the onset of burnout. His complaint focused on the work environment due to intense difficulty interacting with colleagues, attending meetings, presenting events, and socializing with his peers. Unable to refuse commitments anymore due to the imminent possibility of damage to his career and corporate position, he found himself in need of psychotherapeutic intervention. After a careful functional analysis of the situation, it was possible to identify that his current condition of emotional overload resulted from a prolonged period of maladaptive psychological processes in the cognitive ("People will notice how weak I am"), affective (panic attacks and crises of anxiety and fear), attentional (excessive focus on the physiological symptoms of anxiety that exposed his vulnerability), self ("I am weak"), motivational ("I have to avoid exposing myself to embarrassment") and behavioral (he postponed, avoided or fled from any social interaction, both in person and virtually) spheres. The maladaptive functioning kept him in a vicious circle of Frustration, lack of achievement, and depersonalization, with physical and psychological impairment. Tables 12.1 and 12.2 represent the assessment of the situation will be described according to the principles of PBT.

Given the six processes of psychological inflexibility presented by Pedro Table (12.2), there is a compromise of healthy variation in each of the six dimensions. All of them also negatively impacted healthy selection, retention, and context sensitivity processes. They therefore became the target of PBT work. The therapeutic plan included the identification and clarification of life values, mindfulness practices, cognitive defusion strategies, flexibility of self-view, acceptance of experiences, and confrontation of feared situations with consequent expansion of behavioral repertoire. The flexibility of maladaptive processes led to emotional regulation, contributing to the reduction of stress levels, and consequently, recovery of SB. The intervention model was based on the contributions of Acceptance and Commitment Therapy (ACT), a third generation approach of CBT, which has been revealing itself

Table 12.1 Maladaptive version of Pedro's psychological flexibility model

Dimension	Variation	Selection	Retention	Context
Affect	Fear	Alert	Confirms the dysfunctional hypothesis	Maladaptative
Cognition	"They will notice I am nervous"	Protect from the feared event	Confirms the dysfunctional hypothesis	Maladaptative
Attention	Self-focused	Preventive threat monitoring	Confirms the dysfunctional hypothesis	Maladaptative
Self	"I am inadequate"	Prepare for other rejection	Confirms the dysfunctional hypothesis	Maladaptative
Motivation	Don't be rejected	Avoid unwanted consequences	Confirms the dysfunctional hypothesis	Maladaptative
Explicit behavior	Decline invitations to events	Relief from unpleasant sensations	Confirms the dysfunctional hypothesis	Maladaptative

Adaptaded by Hayes et al. (2023b)

Table 12.2 Detailed description of Pedro's psychological inflexibility processes

Dimension	Variation	Inflexibility process
Affect	Fear	Experiential avoidance
Cognition	"They will notice I am nervous"	Cognitive fusion
Attention	Self-focused	Unyielding attention
Self	"I am inadequate"	Self as a concept
Motivation	Don't be rejected	No clarity of values
Explicit behavior	Decline invitations to events	Isolation and reduction of behavioral repertoire

Table 12.3 Description of Pedro's functioning pre- and post-intervention based on processes

Dimension	Maladaptative functioning	Strategies based on processes	Adaptative functioning
Affect	Fear	Acceptance of emotional experiences	Emotional regulation
Cognition	"They will notice I am nervous"	Cognitive defusion	Thought detachments
Atention	Self-focused	Mindfulness practice	Openness to experiences and no judgement
Self	"I am inadequate"	Self as a context	Self-compassion
Motivation	Don't be rejected	Clarification of life values	Attitudes guided by values rather than rules
Explicit behavior	Decline invitation to events	Actions committed to values	Expansion of the behavioral repertoire

as a promising therapeutic for social anxiety disorder (Caletti et al., 2022). Also applied to transdiagnostic cases, ACT aims to promote psychological flexibility and emotional regulation. The following Table 12.3 illustrates the progress of the process-based intervention.

Conclusion

PBT is a very current approach based on the transdiagnostic view. Interventions for stress and for SB present in various clinical complaints, from this perspective, require an expanded view, since this overlap needs to encompass the consideration of common processes between phenomena and diagnoses. Thus, PBT focuses on understanding the dynamics underlying emotional difficulties, providing a more detailed and personalized view to implement effective therapeutic strategies. By focusing on the cognitive, emotional, and behavioral processes common to psychological problems, PBT seeks to understand and intervene in such processes, such as dysfunctional thought patterns, inadequate coping strategies, maladaptive emotional processes, among others. The therapeutic proposal is to work with the identification and modification of these processes, promoting productive and sustainable changes. Based on this model of psychotherapy, the treatment of cases in which there is overlap of stress and/or SB with different clinical conditions can bring results that contribute to improving the quality of life of those who are suffering, as well as allowing therapists to develop broader and more comprehensive interventions that apply to a variety of patients with different complaints.

References

Aderka, I. M., & Hofmann, S. G. (2023). Ansiedade Social. Uma abordagem de tratamento baseada no processo. In D. H. Barlow (Ed.), *Manual Clínico dos Transtornos Psicológicos—Tratamento Passo a Passo* (6ª edição, pp. 169–199). Artmed.

Alarcon, G., Eschleman, K. J., & Bowling, N. A. (2009). Relationships between personality variables and burnout: A meta-analysis. *Work and Stress, 23*, 244–263. https://doi.org/10.1080/02678370903282600

Areosa, J., & Queirós, C. (2020). Burnout. *International Journal on Work Condition, 20*, 71–90.

Barlow, D. (2016). *Manual Clínico dos Transtornos Psicológicos: tratamento passo a passo*. Artmed.

Barlow, D. H., Allen, L. B., & Choate, M. L. (2020). Toward a unified treatment for emotional disorders. In *The neurotic paradox* (Vol. 1, pp. 141–166). Routledge. https://doi.org/10.1016/S0005-7894(04)80036-4

Benevides-Pereira, A. M. T. (2008). *Burnout: quando o trabalho ameaça a saúde do trabalhador*. Casa do Psicólogo.

Bianchi, R., Rolland, J. P., & Salgado, J. F. (2018). Burnout, depression, and borderline personality: A 1,163-participant study. *Frontiers in Psychology, 8*, 2336. https://doi.org/10.3389/fpsyg.2017.02336

Caletti, E., Massimo, C., Magliocca, S., Moltrasio, C., Brambilla, P., & Delvecchio, G. (2022). The role of the acceptance and commitment therapy in the treatment of social anxiety: An updated scoping review. *Journal of Affective Disorders, 310*, 174–182. https://doi.org/10.1016/j.jad.2022.05.008

Chu, B., Marwaha, K., Sanvictores, T., & Ayers, D. (2021). Physiology, stress reaction. In *StatPearls [Internet]*. StatPearls Publishing.

de Aquino, R. L., Barbosa, D. A. F., Santos, L. P., Araújo, N. R. S., Silva, F. F. R., da Cunha Miguel, E., et al. (2023). Análise do Presenteísmo, workaholic, burnout e bornout no contexto do trabalho. *Revista Eletrônica Acervo Científico, 44*, e12867–e12867.

de Ornelas, A. C. C. (2020). Protocolo Unificado para tratamento em transdiagnósticos. In M. R. de Carvalho, E. M. O. Falcone, L. E. N. Malagris, & A. D. Oliva (Orgs.), *Produções em Terapia Cognitivo-comportamental: Integração e Atualização* (pp. 87–97). Artesã.

Eustis, E. H., Gallagher, M. W., Tirpak, J. W., Nauphal, M., Farchione, T. J., & Barlow, D. H. (2020). The Unified Protocol compared with diagnosis-specific protocols for anxiety disorders: 12-month follow-up from a randomized clinical trial. *General Hospital Psychiatry, 67*, 58–61. https://doi.org/10.1016/j.genhosppsych.2020.08.012

Fischer, R., Mattos, P., Teixeira, C., Ganzerla, D. S., Rosa, R. G., & Bozza, F. A. (2020). Association of burnout with depression and anxiety in critical care clinicians in Brazil. *JAMA Network Open, 3*(12), e2030898. https://doi.org/10.1001/jamanetworkopen.2020.30898

Freudenberger, H. J. (1974). Staff burn-out. *Journal of Social Issues, 30*(1), 159–165.

Gallagher, M. W., Sauer-Zavala, S. E., Boswell, J. F., Carl, J. R., Bullis, J., Farchione, T. J., & Barlow, D. H. (2013). The impact of the unified protocol for emotional disorders on quality of life. *International Journal of Cognitive Therapy, 6*(1), 57–72. https://doi.org/10.1521/ijct.2013.6.1.57

Golonka, K., Mojsa-Kaja, J., Blukacz, M., Gawłowska, M., & Marek, T. (2019). Occupational burnout and its overlapping effect with depression and anxiety. *International Journal of Occupational Medicine and Environmental Health, 32*(2), 229–244. https://doi.org/10.13075/ijomeh.1896.01323

Goodman, F. R., Birg, J. A., Daniel, K. E., & Kashdan, T. B. (2023). Stress generation in social anxiety and depression: A two-study community assessment. *Journal of Affective Disorders, 329*, 285–292. https://doi.org/10.1016/j.jad.2023.02.053

Guerra, C. D. S. (2022). *Análise do Burnout como fator de risco para a Ansiedade, Depressão e Qualidade de Vida*. Doctoral dissertation, Universidade da Beira Interior. http://hdl.handle.net/10400.6/13168

Hayes, S. C., & Hofmann, S. G. (2017). The third wave of cognitive behavioral therapy and the rise of process-based care. *World Psychiatry, 16*(3), 245. https://doi.org/10.1002/2Fwps.20442

Hayes, S. C., Hofmann, S. G., Stanton, C. E., Carpenter, J. K., Sanford, B. T., Curtiss, J. E., & Ciarrochi, J. (2019). The role of the individual in the coming era of process-based therapy. *Behaviour Research and Therapy, 117*, 40–53. https://doi.org/10.1016/j.brat.2018.10.005

Hayes, S. C., Hofmann, S. G., & Ciarrochi, J. (2023a). Construindo um sistema diagnóstico baseado em processos: uma perspectiva evolucionista ampliada. In *Para além do DSM: em direção a uma alternativa baseada em processos para diagnóstico e tratamento em saúde mental* (pp. 321–353). Sinopsys.

Hayes, S. C., Hofmann, S. G., & Ciarrochi, J. (2023b). Criando uma alternativa ao diagnóstico sindrômico. In *Para além do DSM: em direção a uma alternativa baseada em processos para diagnóstico e tratamento em saúde mental* (pp. 13–37). Sinopsys.

Hofmann, S. G., & Hayes, S. C. (2018). TCC Moderna CBT: Movendo-se em direção a terapias baseadas em processos. *Revista Brasileira de Terapias Cognitivas, 14*(2), 77–84. http://pepsic.bvsalud.org/scielo.php?pid=S1808-56872018000200003&script=sci_arttext

Hofmann, S. G., & Hayes, S. C. (2019). The future of intervention science: Process-based therapy. *Clinical Psychological Science, 7*(1), 37–50. https://doi.org/10.1177/2167702618772296

Hofmann, S. G., Hayes, S. C., & Lorscheid, D. N. (2023). *Aprendendo a terapia baseada em processos—treinamento de habilidades para a mudança psicológica na prática clínica*. Artmed.

Koutsimani, P., Montgomery, A., & Georganta, K. (2019). The relationship between burnout, depression, and anxiety: A systematic review and meta-analysis. *Frontiers in Psychology, 10*. https://doi.org/10.3389/fpsyg.2019.00284

Lazarus, R. S., & Folkman, S. (1987). Transactional theory and research on emotions and coping. *European Journal of Personality, 1*(3), 141–169.

Lipp, M. E. N. (2000). *Inventário de sintomas de stress para adultos*. Casa do Psicólogo.

Lipp, M. E. N., & Malagris, L. E. N. (2011). Estresse: Aspectos históricos, teóricos e clínicos. In B. Rangé (Org.), *Psicoterapias cognitivo-comportamentais: um diálogo com a psiquiatria* (2a. ed., pp. 617–632). Artmed.

Malagris, L. E. N., & Dias, F. M. (2019). Estresse. In M. Carvalho, L. Malagris, & B. Rangé (Orgs.), *Psicoeducação em terapia cognitivo-comportamental* (pp. 245–256). Sinopsys.

Mansell, W., Rigby, Z., Tai, S., & Lowe, C. (2008). Do current beliefs predict hypomanic symptoms beyond personality style? Factor analysis of the Hypomanic Attitudes and Positive Predictions Inventory (HAPPI) and its association with hypomanic symptoms in a student population. *Journal of Clinical Psychology, 64*(4), 450–465. https://doi.org/10.1002/jclp.20455

Maresca, G., Corallo, F., Catanese, G., Formica, C., & Lo Buono, V. (2022). Coping strategies of healthcare professionals with burnout syndrome: A systematic review. *Medicina, 58*(2), 327.

Maslach, C., & Jackson, S. E. (1981). The measurement of experienced burnout. *Journal of Occupational Behavior, 2*(2), 99–113.

Maslach, C., & Jackson, S. E. (1986). *Maslach burnout inventory*. Consulting Psychologist Press.

Mesquita, V. S. M., & Malagris, L. E. N. (2020). Síndrome de Burnout em residentes multiprofissionais em saúde de um hospital universitário. *Revista da Sociedade Brasileira de Psicologia Hospitalar, 23*(2), 65–76.

World Health Organization (OMS). (2019). *ICD-11 reference guide*. OMS, Disponível em inglês em: https://icd.who.int/icd11refguide/en/index.html. Acesso em 02 de janeiro de 2024.

Queirós, C., Borges, E., & Abreu, M. (2019). Ansiedade, Engagement e Burnout em enfermeiros. In *International Congress of Occupational Health Nursing: Proceedings*.

Selye, H. (1965). *Stress: a tensão da vida*. Ibrasa.

Selye, H. (1976). *The stress of life*. Mcgraw-Hill.

Skodol, A. E., Gunderson, J. G., McGlashan, T. H., Dyck, I. R., Stout, R. L., Bender, D. S., et al. (2002). Functional impairment in patients with schizotypal, borderline, avoidant, or obsessive-compulsive personality disorder. *American Journal Psychiatry, 159*, 276–283. https://doi.org/10.1176/appi.ajp.159.2.276

Straub, O. (2014). Estresse e Saúde. In O. Straub (Ed.), *Psicologia da Saúde. Uma abordagem biopsicossocial* (3rd ed., pp. 75–140). Artmed.

Taris, T. W., Le Blanc, P. M., Schaufeli, W. B., & Schreurs, P. J. (2005). Are there causal relationships between the dimensions of the Maslach Burnout Inventory? A review and two longitudinal tests. *Work & Stress, 19*(3), 238–255.

Tavares, M. L., Soares-Fortunato, J. M., & Leite-Moreira, A. F. (2000). Stress Respostas fisiológicas e fisiopatológicas. *Revista Portuguesa de Psicossomática, 2*(2), 51–65.

Xu, C., Xu, Y., Xu, S., Zhang, Q., Liu, X., Shao, Y., et al. (2020). Cognitive reappraisal and the association between perceived stress and anxiety symptoms in COVID-19 isolated people. *Frontiers in Psychiatry, 11*, 858.

Chapter 13
Process-Based Therapy

Wilson Vieira Melo, Jan Luiz Leonardi, Débora C. Fava, Ramiro Figueiredo Catelan, Katia Caetano, and André Luiz Moreno

Introduction

The dominant psychiatric paradigm defines a mental disorder as "a syndrome characterized by clinically significant disturbance in an individual's cognition, emotion regulation, or behavior that reflects a dysfunction in the psychological, biological, or developmental processes underling mental functioning" (APA, 2022, p. 20). This definition reflects a medical illness model which see clients' symptoms as the expression of latent diseases.

For many years, government agencies adopted that paradigm and allocated funding to randomized clinical trials (RCT) to assess specific protocols targeting psychiatric syndromes. This tailored clinical science, and for almost five decades research in the field has developed protocols for syndromes and assessed them via RCT (Thompson-Hollands et al., 2014).

Cognitive and Behavioral Therapy (CBT) was significantly impacted by that, and a vast list of specialized treatment protocols was developed for treating several disorders in the last decades. CBT was solidified as the most empirically validated therapeutic approach as there was solid data regarding its efficacy (Hofmann et al., 2012).

W. V. Melo (✉) · D. C. Fava · R. F. Catelan
Porto Alegre, RS, Brazil

J. L. Leonardi
Catanduva, SP, Brazil

K. Caetano
Barra, Bahia, Brazil

A. L. Moreno
Uberaba, MG, Brazil

A. C. Ornelas (ed.), *Transdiagnostic Approaches in Cognitive Behavioral Therapy*, https://doi.org/10.1007/978-3-031-63494-9_13

The proliferation of specialized protocols hindered the scalability and accessibility of comprehensive care though. Critically, the protocol for syndrome-based model tends to overlook idiographic aspects such as comorbidity, client diversity, and individual client's nuances and needs, procedural specificity, and the processes of change. Thus, there's a pressing need to integrate a more process-oriented perspective to enhance therapeutic effectiveness and responsiveness to individual needs (Hayes et al., 2020).

Mental health and intervention science fields have been changing towards a new process-based paradigm that is individual-focused and evidence-based. This model prioritizes targeting core change processes anchored in empirically testable theories. Rather than addressing latent disease entities through standardized evidence-based intervention protocols, the process-based model increasingly emphasizes understanding and assessing the specific processes conducive to meaningful therapeutic change (Hayes & Hofmann, 2021).

Process-based therapy (PBT) is a new paradigm in the evidence-based intervention science. It focuses on processes that are both contextually specific and substantiated by evidence, aiming to reduce distress and bolster individual well-being. Differently from protocol-based intervention approach, PBT emphasizes processes grounded in theoretical frameworks and backed by empirical data, acknowledging their essential contribution to achieving favorable treatment results (Hayes & Hofmann, 2021; Hofmann & Hayes, 2019).

In the PBT paradigm practitioners are prompted to explore the functional relationships between a client's challenges and the contexts in which they manifest. This approach focuses on the process of change to conceptualize the development and persistence of clients' clinical demands. By gaining insights into these functional connections, therapists can then work towards adapting and refining clients' network (Hayes & Hofmann, 2018).

Addressing individual client's complexities through functional analysis and case formulation rather than treating syndromes through standard protocols is not new and has historical roots in behavior therapy. However, PBT has expanded and further developed the initial tradition and incorporated an empirical complex network approach based on research from the last decades. Several process-based interventions such as acceptance and commitment therapy, dialectical behavioral therapy, mindfulness-based cognitive therapy and functional analytic psychotherapy have been accumulating robust data on the process of change, mediators and moderators that can help therapists to build a tailored intervention for a client (Hayes & Hofmann, 2018).

Answering questions as which processes should be addressed with a given client, considering her/his unique goals, history, and context is the core feature of PBT. The aim is to elucidate how these processes can be modified in the most efficient and effective way through evidence-based interventions tailored to individual needs and contexts (Hofmann & Hayes, 2019).

PBT emerges as a versatile, philosophy-driven approach centered on the processes underlying therapeutic change. Over the past decades, PBT science has studied several processes that influence outcomes. This research can assist clinicians in determining which procedures might be most beneficial for targeting specific processes for a specific client at a particular moment. Furthermore, PBT underscores the critical importance of understanding and emphasizing processes of change, with an emphasis on moderation and mediation, enriching both behavioral and cognitive therapeutic practices (Hayes & Hofmann, 2018, 2021).

Problems with DSM and ICD

In 1993, the Division 12 of the American Psychological Association (APA) established a task force with the goal of identifying empirically supported treatments (ESTs). This initiative had multiple objectives: developing training guidelines for future therapists, providing ongoing education for current practitioners, promoting the integration of ESTs into health plans, and enhancing public awareness of psychotherapy's effectiveness (Chambless, 1993). To identify ESTs, the task force set forth three criteria: firstly, the intervention must be manualized, detailing its conceptual, structural, and technical aspects; secondly, it should address specific clinical issues, predominantly those outlined in the Diagnostic and Statistical Manual of Mental Disorders (DSM; American Psychiatric Association, 2022), so that it would not simply be classified as an EST, but rather, for example, as an EST for major depressive disorder or an EST for borderline personality disorder; thirdly, its efficacy must have been established through diverse research, evidenced by at least two randomized clinical trials or nine single-subject experiments. In 2015, Division 12 revised this third criterion, shifting the focus from a specified number of studies to the use of systematic reviews, which summarizes the evidence of efficacy of a given intervention for a given clinical condition, for assessing an intervention's efficacy for specific clinical conditions (Tolin et al., 2015).

Despite their advantages, manualized ESTs have limitations. One of them is that most ESTs focus on DSM-defined psychopathologies. While DSM categories offer a lot of benefits, such as diagnostic reliability, risk factor research, prognosis study, communication between professionals, and treatment research, they are not without issues. Key concerns include:

Rigid Categories: The DSM classifies psychological suffering into more or less rigid categories, but behavioral, cognitive, and emotional problems vary in degree, rather than being merely present or absent. Therefore, the division between "pathological" and "healthy" is not always clear.

Diagnostic Heterogeneity: Many traditional diagnoses can be exceedingly varied, leading to uncertainty about their true meaning. For instance, borderline personality disorder can be diagnosed based on 256 different symptom combinations, and post-traumatic stress disorder has over 636,120 possible symptom combinations.

High Comorbidity: The co-occurrence of multiple psychopathologies is more common than singular diagnoses (Kessler et al., 2005), challenging the notion of distinct diagnostic categories.

Moreover, some scholars (cf. Reed et al., 2006) argue that diagnoses often fail to capture the unique aspects and contextual backgrounds of clients' issues. Others (e.g., Bohart et al., 1998) believe that diagnoses are unnecessary for client description, advocating for personalized treatment approaches rather than labeling individuals based on shared characteristics. Additionally, many clients exhibit symptoms like anxiety, depression, drug use, and personality shifts that do not meet the full criteria for a diagnosis, while others seek therapy for non-DSM issues, such as challenges related to major life changes, such as moving to a new city, starting a new job, or transitioning to retirement, guidance on making significant lifestyle changes, such as adopting a healthier lifestyle or managing work-life balance, coping with the death of a loved one, end of a relationship, or loss of a cherished pet, addressing existential questions, etc. (Fava & Mangelli, 2001; Stirman et al., 2003; Westen & Arkowitz-Westen, 1998).

What Is a Process?

In psychology, particularly in PBT, a process is understood as a series of events known to influence a person's well-being. These processes can be direct, such as the impact of regular exercise on well-being, or indirect, such as how witnessing someone's healthy habits might inspire one's own health choices. Their complexity is highlighted by their simultaneous occurrence and interaction within a person, affecting their overall well-being in diverse ways. Moreover, they can have both positive and negative impacts. For example, some processes might contribute to a person's distress or dysfunction, while others might facilitate adaptive functioning and resilience. The individuality of these processes, influenced by personal context and life experiences, underscores the dynamic nature of human behavior and well-being (Hofmann et al., 2021).

Processes have crucial evolutionary components, which rebounds their adaptative nature. They are not static, evolving over time and adapting to new circumstances and information. Evolutionary lenses are elementary in understanding how processes can be modified or optimized in various contexts, whether in nature, technology, or human behavior. The adaptability of processes indicates their capacity to change in response to external stimuli or internal feedback mechanisms, demonstrating a level of complexity and sophistication in how processes are structured and function.

An evolutionary framework is seen as a critical component for PBT's processes concept, which recognizes the importance of evolution in understanding human behavior and psychological processes. This approach applies evolutionary principles like variation, selection, and retention to psychological processes, considering them within the context of a person's environment and history. PBT's evolutionary perspective helps in identifying and organizing key biopsychosocial processes that are functionally important to mental health and human well-being. It emphasizes the dynamic and adaptive nature of psychological processes, considering how these processes have developed and evolved over time in response to environmental and internal factors. This evolutionary framework provides a more nuanced understanding of mental health issues, moving beyond traditional syndrome-based diagnoses to a more comprehensive, individualized approach (Hayes et al., 2020).

Further diving into the nuances of therapeutic processes, processes are characterized by specific qualities that guide clinical interventions. These processes are theory-based, dynamic, progressive, contextually bound, and part of a multilevel system. Each of these qualities contributes to the effectiveness and applicability of therapeutic interventions. For instance, a theory-based process is grounded in a clear understanding of the relationships among various events, leading to testable predictions. Dynamic processes involve feedback loops and non-linear changes, reflecting the complexity of human psychology. The progressive nature of processes indicates the necessity of sequencing them appropriately to achieve therapeutic goals. Being contextually bound, these processes are adaptable and relevant to the individual's specific circumstances. Finally, the multilevel aspect of processes acknowledges that they can operate at different levels of human functioning, from individual thoughts and emotions to broader social and cultural influences (Hofmann et al., 2021).

What Is a Procedure?

Traditional therapeutic approaches aim at mitigating mental disorder-derived suffering. The current evidence-based psychological practice paradigm, grounded in the syndrome model of mental illness, proposes that there should be specific treatment protocols to address each mental disorder. To address the limitations of this model, Hayes and Hofmann (2018) suggest that therapists should learn procedures previously described in the evidence-based psychotherapy literature to address processes instead of concentrating on treating mental disorders with syndrome-focused protocols. Procedures refer to specific therapeutic techniques or actions tailored to address the unique psychological processes of an individual. These procedures are not one-size-fits-all but are chosen and applied based on a thorough understanding of the individual's specific psychological processes, instead of addressing particular mental disorders. This personalized approach would ensure that the therapy would be more effective and relevant to the individual's needs.

Procedures, according to the PBT approach, are dynamic and adaptable. As the therapy progresses and as more is understood about the individual's psychological makeup, the procedures can be adjusted. This flexibility allows for a more responsive and effective therapeutic process, where interventions are continuously fine-tuned to meet the evolving needs of the individual. Furthermore, PBT posits an integrative perspective for procedures, combining elements from various therapeutic traditions and models. This integration is guided by a deep understanding of how different processes operate and interact within an individual. By drawing from a diverse set of therapeutic tools and techniques, PBT offers a comprehensive approach to mental health treatment (Hofmann et al., 2021).

One of the procedures described in the PBT literature is cognitive restructuring (Wenzel, 2018), which might be used to address negative thought patterns in a client suffering from anxiety. The therapist would assess how these thought patterns contribute to the client's anxiety and tailor cognitive restructuring techniques specifically to address these patterns. This could involve teaching the client to identify and challenge irrational beliefs, fostering a more adaptive way of thinking. Another procedure might involve emotion regulation training to help a client manage intense emotions (Aldao & Plate, 2018). This could include teaching the client to identify specific emotions, understand the situations that trigger these emotions, and develop strategies for responding to these emotions in a healthy way. For instance, if a client struggles with anger, they might learn techniques to recognize the early signs of anger and use coping strategies like deep breathing or mindfulness to manage their response. By doing that, a therapist would empower clients to handle their emotions more effectively, leading to improved mental health and well-being. These examples illustrate how procedures are both specific to the individual's needs and grounded in broader psychological principles.

Network Model/Extended Evolutionary Metamodel (EEMM)

To address the specificity of each client functioning it is important to recognize that processes are connected in a network system. With this understanding, therapists can make more informed choices about psychotherapeutic procedures. To illustrate network thinking and the Extended Evolutionary Metamodel (EEMM) (Hofmann et al., 2021), various fields beyond psychology use network models to explain relationships between components. In PBT, the authors have created a way to explain the relationship between processes using boxes to represent events or the functioning of a person, and arrows to illustrate the connection between them. These relationships can be simple or complex, and the arrows depict the sequence and the impact of one event on another. A simple relationship is illustrated in the following example of 45-year-old patient named Olga (see Fig. 13.1).

Following the event of experiencing psychological abuse from her husband and first boyfriend, Olga developed difficulty in making decisions for her personal life. At the same time, after many years of enduring the abuse, we understand that there is a bidirectional communication between the boxes (see Fig. 13.2).

Due to the difficulty in making decisions, Olga is unable to interrupt the continuity of abuse, as various possibilities (such as reporting to the police, seeking a divorce, activating a support network, etc.) seem to generate a state of fear and confusion, perpetuating this difficulty. In this sense, we observe a complex network

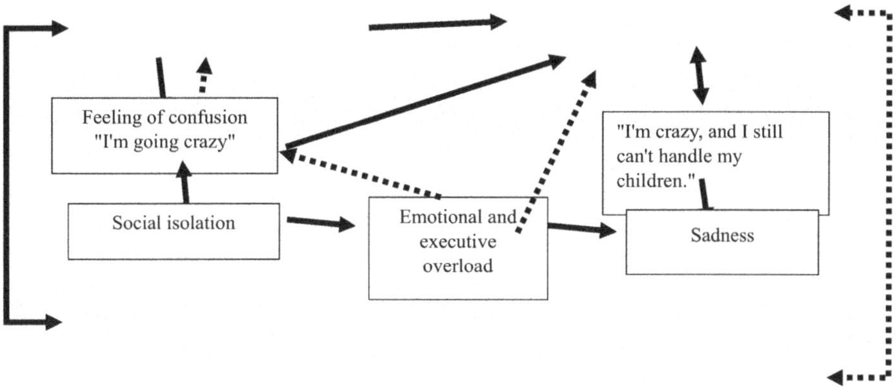

Fig. 13.1 Relationship between processes

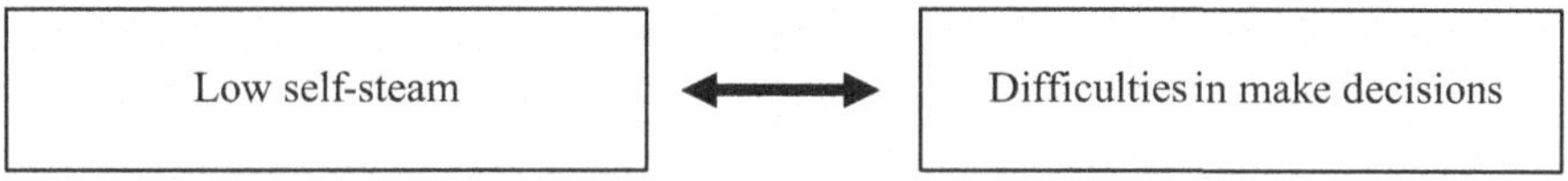

Fig. 13.2 Bidirectional communication

relationship, in which a feedback loop has been established. When a person develops this loop continuously over an extended period, they tend to become more resistant to change, triggering new events and processes in the network.

These feedback loops become even more complex when we include other elements that illustrate in more detail the functioning of the patient. Typically, these other elements form sub-networks within this broader network (History of psychological abuse—Difficulty in making decisions).

In Olga's example, it is possible to observe two main sub-networks (see Fig. 13.3). In the first one, the history of abuse leads the patient to isolate herself from social life, living solely for her husband and children, causing emotional and executive overload (many demands from home and children solely on her). This impact reinforces the feeling of confusion and of going crazy that psychological abuse directly caused.

Each element in the network is crucial for us to understand which processes are more responsible for the patient's symptoms. This analysis attempts to facilitate the understanding of the patient's functioning, but still relies on the therapist's clinical understanding and reasoning.

For example, if in Olga's life history, she has had academic difficulties and trouble making decisions in adolescence, this process likely has a more central characteristic in her life. In this regard, she could benefit from cognitive rehabilitation in conjunction with psychotherapy, or consider medication, thinking that it might be related to a probable Attention Deficit/Hyperactivity Disorder. However, if the "social isolation" event has a significant impact currently, contributing to feelings of

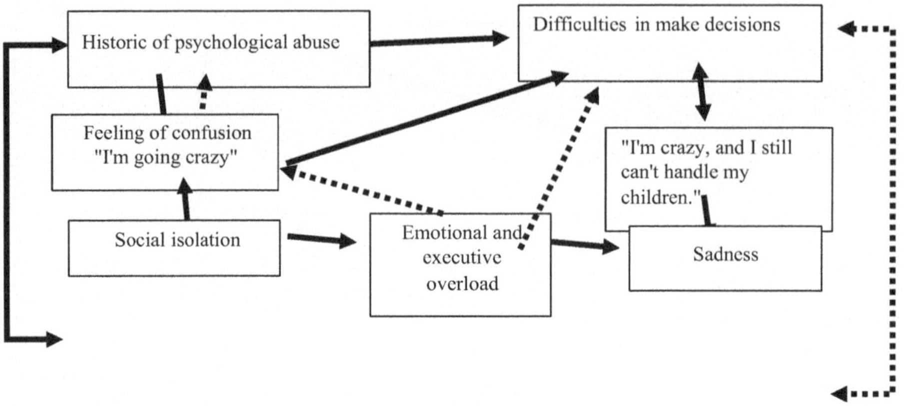

Fig. 13.3 Client's process

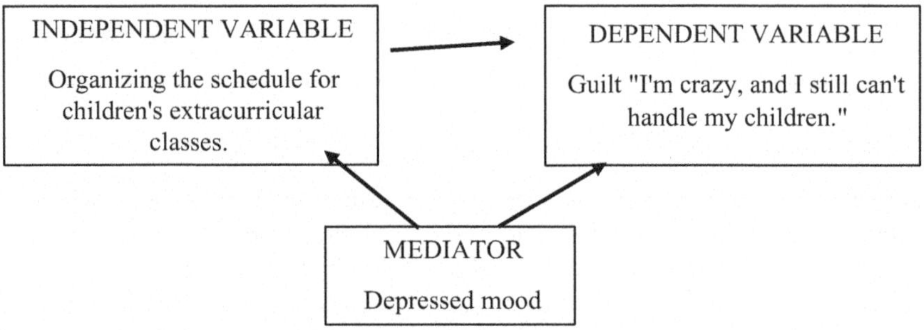

Fig. 13.4 Mediator, independent variable and dependent variable

loneliness, overload, and depressive symptoms, Olga may benefit from an intervention that initially focuses on improving relationships beyond the family nucleus.

In Olga's case, from any perspective we look at her system and network, we find a complex case that changes in one element will affect all other processes. This is the point where the clinician needs to be very careful to avoid iatrogenic effects in psychotherapy.

Knowing more precisely which processes should be targeted for change in psychotherapy requires an understanding of the mediating effect that one component can have on another. The 'mediator' is the mechanism through which the independent variable (IV) influences the dependent variable (DV), our target for change (see Fig. 13.4).

In a broad sense, we can understand that the Dependent Variable (VD) involving inappropriate self-blame, which is a psychotherapeutic target, is influenced by the Independent Variable (VI) "organizing the schedule." The current depressed mood acts as a mediator in this sub-network system. Within a patient's network system, it's possible to find various mediators, DVs, and IVs, depending on the perspective and the part of this subsystem we want to analyze.

Evolutionary Extended Meta Model (EEMM)

The Extended Evolutionary Metamodel (EEMM) is a proposal that organizes relevant information for change processes, aiming for unified communication among clinicians. Additionally, it serves as a prescriptive guide for selecting interventions available in the scientific literature that best apply to specific processes of each patient. As complex as it may be to understand all human processes, PBT has gathered some that can sufficiently explain the patient's functioning. Therefore, the components cognition, emotion, attention, self, motivation, and behavior are part of the EEMM.

Furthermore, beyond the psychological level, the authors emphasize the importance of the biophysiological and sociocultural levels. For each of the processes, it is crucial to identify evolutionary aspects that best explain the symptom or functioning. Table 13.1 shows the components of the EEMM and recognizes the existence of an adaptive presentation in addition to the maladaptive one.

The cognitive dimension relates to how a person thinks and relates to their thoughts. In large part, Cognitive-Behavioral Therapy assists the clinician in identifying these thought patterns, attributional style, and cognitive distortions through techniques such as Socratic questioning, for example.

The affective dimension relates to how a person feels their emotions and how they relate to them. "Experiential avoidance," known as a process in Acceptance and Commitment Therapy (ACT), is an example of how to deal with emotions, i.e., by distancing oneself from them. On the other hand, "acceptance" is a process that allows the individual to observe their emotions and internal reactions without necessarily trying to get rid of them or fuse with them.

The attentional dimension explains how patients shift the direction and focus of their internal and external experiences. It is challenging to separate these dimensions, but this is done for pedagogical reasons. We emphasize this because this dimension communicates directly with the cognitive dimension and may seem, in some cases, overlapping. A more rigid, more scattered, or hyper-focused attention on the past or the future can be examples of variation in this dimension.

The Self dimension essentially refers to patients' beliefs—what they think about themselves, which can be adaptive or maladaptive. The self reflects a sequence of learnings about oneself that takes a self-amplifying form. Moreover, maladaptive forms of the Self often bring short-term gains, such as relief, but in the long run, they maintain maladaptive functioning and suffering.

The motivational dimension concerns the source of motivation for change, such as acting based on values, having goals and planning, but it can also refer to factors that motivate the persistence of the problem, such as complacency and apparent indifference.

The behavioral dimension refers to how the individual behaves, how they act in various situations. Generally, in a maladaptive manner, the expressed behavior is governed by the set of beliefs and other components of the EEMM. Similarly, manifest dysfunctional behavior keeps the other processes active.

Table 13.1 Olga's extended evolutionary metamodel

	Variation	Selection	Retention
Affective	Guilt, sadness	Keeps her trapped in her dependent functioning	When she feels guilty, the husband "shows her" how she needs him
Cognitive	"I can't handle it." "I'm confused." "I'm crazy."	The function of these thoughts is to maintain the marriage, given that she has only this relationship	These thoughts keep her a victim of psychological abuse and prevent her from confronting autonomy and independence
Attentional	Ruminative thoughts related to self-blame and inadequacy appear	Focusing on Olga's distorted past confirms thoughts that make her feel guilty for what happens in her life	This direction of attention towards past events reinforces the idea that she will not be enough, feeding a sense of hopelessness in herself, which can impact motivation for change
Self	Incapacity Insufficiency	By seeing herself as incapable or insufficient, she maintains her abusive marriage	By keeping her marriage as it is, she avoids the discomfort of change and the pursuit of a more meaningful life
Motivation	Complacency	Olga acts based on what is important or right for her husband	She maintains the cycle that reinforces her own functioning and the current depression
	Love for her children	Olga is very interested in doing the best for her children	It can be an important component to motivate change and be an assertive example of self-respect for her children
Behavior	Difficulty in taking prompt action Slowness in performing household tasks Cries and complains about herself	Acting in this way, Olga maintains her belief system of insufficiency and her feelings of guilt	Being in an abusive relationship where the husband reinforces her need to depend on him maintains the dysfunctional cycle

Not all parts of the EEMM need to be filled in. The idea is not to fit the client into it but to use it to better understand the client. The "biophysiological" and sociocultural dimensions establish a context for the six dimensions. In the biophysiological dimension, clinical, genetic, or physiological aspects of the client, as well as diseases, among others, may be related or somehow explaining or contributing to the other dimensions. In the sociocultural dimension, aspects related to family and other transgenerational contributions can help explain the functioning of the patient and the origin and maintenance of this. Just as issues related to culture, historical, and religious aspects can also be understood in this dimension.

Within the EEMM, the contextual dimension plays a crucial role in a comprehensive understanding of the individual. This dimension encompasses the biopsychosocial aspects shaping the patient's experience, incorporating biological, psychological, and social elements. On the biological front, issues related to physical health and genetics are considered, providing insights into potential contributions to psychological functioning. Psychologically, the context includes the patient's cognitive, emotional, and motivational history, examining how these factors interact and influence their internal processes. In the social realm, the EEMM takes into account factors such as family relationships, cultural influences, and the social environment, emphasizing the significance of these contexts in the origin and maintenance of behavioral and emotional patterns. This contextual dimension within the EEMM allows for a more holistic understanding of the individual, integrating various elements contributing to their unique experience and guiding the formulation of more effective therapeutic strategies tailored to the specific needs of the client.

Conclusion

This chapter aimed to present the historical and theoretical basis of Process-based Therapy (PBT), a new approach to understanding how evidence-based practice could be understood in a broader context than the current guidelines. PBT strengthens how each individual mental health problem, and therefore treatment, should be highlighted as the focus of psychological interventions. Also, PBT offers a clearer hypothesis of how evolutionary perspectives should be considered in the conceptualization of clients' problems and symptoms.

As with every new paradigm, PBT's theory must develop to solve some underlying questions still unanswered. For example, PBT proposes an integration of nomothetic and idiographic data to consolidate itself as an evidence-based practice. However, it is still unclear how this integration would be made, considering that the triangulation of first-person data with third-person data is a historical problem of experimental psychology. Another question, for example, refers to how PBT would advocate in favor of one theoretical base instead of another. Despite a concise and clear definition of what processes and procedures are, it is important to clarify that some of these specific concepts could be related to different approaches in psychology and, therefore, could be an important source of misunderstanding.

Moreover, it is important to highlight that data from clinical studies using PBT as a primary source of case conceptualization and intervention planning is still sparse and outnumbered. All existing data up to this date come from experts' comments or case studies, which are considered a weak source of evidence to support evidence-based practice. It is expected that more data, coming from different methodologies, will enlighten the theoretical claim of PBT as a strong lens to evidence-based practice.

Nevertheless, PBT has already granted some importance in the psychotherapy field while pointing out some historical problems regarding evidence-based practice as it has been structured over the years and offering a concise and bright model to conceptualize cases, plan interventions, and assess patients' results. It is expected that further theoretical advances combined with clinical data from broader methodological sources clarify what role PBT will play in the psychotherapy field in the years to come.

References

Aldao, A., & Plate, A. J. (2018). Coping and emotion regulation. In S. C. Hayes & S. G. Hofmann (Eds.), *Process-based CBT: The science and core clinical competencies of cognitive behavioral therapy* (pp. 261–271). New Harbinger Publications, Inc.

American Psychiatric Association. (2022). *Diagnostic and statistical manual of mental disorders* (5th ed., text rev.) (DSM-5-TR). American Psychiatric Publications, Inc.

Bohart, A. D., O'Hara, M., & Leitner, L. M. (1998). Empirically violated treatments: Disenfranchisement of humanistic and other psychotherapies. *Psychotherapy Research, 8*, 141–157.

Chambless, D. L. (1993). *Task force on promotion and dissemination of psychological procedures: A report adopted by the Division 12 Board*. American Psychological Association.

Fava, G. A., & Mangelli, L. (2001). Assessment of subclinical symptoms and psychological well-being in depression. *European Archive of Psychiatry and Clinical Neuroscience, 251*, 47–52.

Hayes, S. C., & Hofmann, S. G. (Eds.). (2018). *Process-based CBT: The science and core clinical competencies of cognitive behavioral therapy*. New Harbinger Publications, Inc.

Hayes, S. C., & Hofmann, S. G. (2021). "Third-wave" cognitive and behavioral therapies and the emergence of a process-based approach to intervention in psychiatry. *World Psychiatry, 20*(3), 363–375.

Hayes, S. C., Hofmann, S. G., & Ciarrochi, J. (2020). A process-based approach to psychological diagnosis and treatment: The conceptual and treatment utility of an extended evolutionary meta model. *Clinical Psychology Review, 82*, 101908.

Hofmann, S. G., & Hayes, S. C. (2019). The future of intervention science: Process-based therapy. *Clinical Psychology Science, 7*(1), 37–50.

Hofmann, S. G., Asnaani, A., Vonk, J. J., Sawyer, A. T., & Fang, A. (2012). The efficacy of cognitive behavioral therapy: A review of meta-analyses. *Cognitive Therapy and Research, 36*, 427–440.

Hofmann, S. G., Hayes, S. C., & Lorscheid, D. N. (2021). *Learning process-based therapy: A skills training manual for targeting the core processes of psychological change in clinical practice*. Context Press.

Kessler, R. C., Chiu, W. T., Demler, O., et al. (2005). Prevalence, severity, and comorbidity of 12-month DSM-IV disorders in the National Comorbidity Survey Replication. *Archives of General Psychiatry, 62*, 617–627.

Reed, G. M., Kihlstrom, J. F., & Messer, S. B. (2006). What qualifies as evidence of effective practice? In J. C. Norcross, L. E. Beutler, & R. F. Levant (Orgs.), *Evidence-based practices in mental health: Debate and dialogue on the fundamental questions* (pp. 13–55). American Psychological Association.

Stirman, S. W., DeRubeis, R. J., CritsChristoph, P., & Brody, P. E. (2003). Are samples in randomized controlled trials of psychotherapy representative of community outpatients? A new methodology and initial findings. *Journal of Consulting and Clinical Psychology, 71*(6), 963–972.

Thompson-Hollands, J., Sauer-Zavala, S., & Balrow, D. H. (2014). CBT and the future of personalized treatment: A proposal. *Depression and Anxiety, 31*, 909–911.

Tolin, D. F., McKay, D., Forman, E. M., Klonsky, E. D., & Thombs, B. D. (2015). Empirically supported treatment: Recommendations for a new model. *Clinical Psychology: Science and Practice, 22*(4), 1–22.

Wenzel, A. (2018). Cognitive reappraisal. In S. C. Hayes & S. G. Hofmann (Eds.), *Process-based CBT: The science and core clinical competencies of cognitive behavioral therapy* (pp. 325–337). New Harbinger Publications, Inc.

Westen, D., & Arkowitz-Westen, L. (1998). Limitations of Axis II in diagnosing personality pathology in clinical practice. *American Journal of Psychiatry, 155*(12), 1767–1771.

Chapter 14
Application of Cognitive Behavioral Therapy Associated with Pharmacotherapy for Anxious and Depressive Disorders

Bruno A. Franco, Laiana A. Quagliato, and Antonio E. Nardi

Introduction

Anxiety and depressive disorders in clinical practice require effective therapeutic measures to control symptoms and thus guarantee patients' quality of life. This chapter aims to discuss the theoretical foundations of diagnoses and forms of treatment, highlighting how Cognitive Behavioral Therapy (CBT) and pharmacotherapy are fundamental for the treatment of these disorders.

There is evidence that validates CBT in identifying and modifying negative thought patterns, while pharmacotherapy aims at symptomatic stabilization. In this chapter we will focus on concepts about disorders, their individual treatments and the integration between these and treatment methods, highlighting how their combined application can enhance therapeutic results in the treatment of these disorders.

Anxiety Disorders

Anxiety disorders represent one of the psychiatric conditions that most affect people around the world. In 2019, around 301 million people had an anxiety disorder according to data from the World Health Organization. Regarding their etiology, the authors highlight the interaction of genetic, neurobiological, and environmental factors in the development of these disorders.

This group of diagnoses presents a variety of clinical manifestations, which according to Sadock and Sadock (2007), include anxious symptoms such as fear, worry, and excessive apprehension, which will generate behavioral consequences, causing suffering and harm to the individual's quality of life for a specified time.

B. A. Franco · L. A. Quagliato · A. E. Nardi (✉)
IPUB/UFRJ, Rio de Janeiro, Brazil

A. C. Ornelas (ed.), *Transdiagnostic Approaches in Cognitive Behavioral Therapy*, https://doi.org/10.1007/978-3-031-63494-9_14

Table 14.1 Generalized Anxiety Disorder criteria

Diagnostic criteria for Generalized Anxiety Disorder according to DSM-V:
A. Excessive anxiety and worry, present most days for at least 6 months, about a series of events or activities
B. The individual finds it difficult to control the worry
C. Anxiety and worry are associated with three (or more) of the following six symptoms:
1. Restlessness or feeling of having "nerves on edge"
2. Fatigability
3. Difficulty concentrating or "blank" sensations in the mind
4. Irritability
5. Muscle tension
6. Sleep disorders (difficulty falling asleep, difficulty staying asleep, or poor sleep)
D. Anxiety, worry, or physical symptoms cause clinically significant distress or impairment in social, occupational, or other important areas of life functioning
E. The disturbance is not attributable to the physiological effects of a substance (e.g., a drug of abuse or a medication) or another medical condition
F. The disturbance is not better explained by a mental disorder

Within the group of anxiety disorders, some specific diagnoses are differentiated according to their individual clinical manifestations. According to criteria in the Diagnostic and Statistical Manual of Mental Disorders (DSM V) (2014), examples of the main diagnoses are generalized anxiety disorder, panic disorder, social anxiety disorder, agoraphobia, and specific phobia.

The symptoms of these diagnoses differ in the types of objects or situations that induce fear, anxiety, or avoidance behavior and the content of thoughts, taking as an example the distinct diagnoses: generalized anxiety disorder and panic disorder, described in Tables 14.1 and 14.2 respectively.

The understanding of the symptomatic and etiological diversity of these disorders allows the discussion of more individualized therapeutic approaches, with Cognitive-Behavioral Therapy being one of the forms of treatment, which offers specific techniques to modify dysfunctional cognitive patterns of anxious conditions. Furthermore, pharmacotherapy plays a significant role in symptomatic relief, especially in more severe cases.

Depressive Disorders

Depressive disorders present themselves as a group of mental conditions that profoundly affect emotional well-being and social functionality, causing a significant impact on the quality of life of affected individuals, according to data from the World Health Organization, approximately 280 million people in the world worldwide were diagnosed with depression in 2023.

Table 14.2 Panic disorder criteria

Diagnostic criteria for panic disorder according to DSM-V:
A. Presence of recurring and unexpected panic attacks. A panic attack is defined as a sudden period of fear intense or severe discomfort that peaks within minutes and is associated with four (or more) of the following symptoms:
1. Palpitations, fast heartbeat, or irregular heart rhythm
2. Tremors
3. Feeling of shortness of breath or suffocation
4. Choking sensations
5. Chest pain or discomfort
6. Nausea or abdominal discomfort
7. Feeling dizzy, unsteady, lightheaded, or faint
8. Depersonalization (feelings of unreality) or derealization (feeling of being in an imaginary world)
9. Fear of losing control or going crazy
10. Fear to die
11. Chills or hot flashes
B. At least one of the panic attacks has been followed by a month (or more) of one (or more) of the following symptoms:
1. Persistent worry about the possibility of having more panic attacks or their consequences (e.g., losing control, having a heart attack, going crazy)
2. Significant changes in behavior related to panic attacks (e.g., avoiding triggering situations)
C. Panic attacks are not attributable to the physiological effects of a substance (e.g., a drug of abuse, medication) or another general medical condition (e.g., hyperthyroidism or cardiovascular disease)
D. The disturbance is not better explained by another mental disorder

The etiology of depressive disorders is multifactorial, involving interaction between genetic, neurobiological, and environmental factors. Family history, traumatic events, neurochemical imbalances, and everyday stressors contribute to individual vulnerability, increasing the risk of developing these conditions.

The clinical presentation according to DSM V, the depressive episode presents symptoms that include depressed mood, anhedonia, changes in appetite and sleep, fatigue, feelings of guilt or worthlessness, and difficulty concentrating, symptoms that are important for the diagnosis of a major depressive episode, which is described in Table 14.3.

The therapeutic approach to depression, as well as anxiety disorders, is diverse. Pharmacotherapy, with the use of antidepressants, is often prescribed to alleviate symptoms, but psychosocial interventions and strategies to promote well-being, such as physical exercise and healthy eating, are forms of non-pharmacological treatment that also play an important role for symptomatic control, as well as cognitive behavioral therapy.

Table 14.3 Major Depressive Disorder criteria

Diagnostic criteria for Major Depressive Episode according to DSM-V:
1. Depressed mood most of the day, almost every day, reported subjectively or observed by others
2. Marked reduction in interest or pleasure in all or almost all activities for most of the day, almost every day
3. Significant weight loss or gain (or decrease or increase in appetite) without being on a diet, or decrease or increase in appetite almost every day
4. Insomnia or hypersomnia almost every day
5. Psychomotor agitation or retardation almost every day (observed by others, not merely subjective feelings of restlessness or slowing)
6. Fatigue or loss of energy almost every day
7. Feeling of worthlessness or excessive or inappropriate guilt almost every day
8. Diminished ability to think, concentrate, or make decisions almost every day
9. Frequent thoughts of death, recurrent suicidal ideation without a specific plan, suicide attempt, or a specific plan to commit suicide

Cognitive-Behavioral Therapy (CBT)

Cognitive-behavioral therapy is a therapeutic approach widely used in clinical psychology and according to Cuijpers et al. (2016a), 75% of patients prefer psychotherapy to the use of medication. As described by Knapp and Beck (2008), Aaron Beck, founder of the concepts of cognitive therapy, states that our thoughts influence our emotions and behaviors, and CBT aims to identify and modify dysfunctional cognitive patterns to promote positive and lasting changes.

This therapy proposal is based on collaboration between therapist and patient to explore and understand the automatic cognitions that shape emotional reactions. Beck's cognitive behavioral therapy approach is structured and focused on the present, focusing on specific goals and practical skills to deal with immediate challenges as demonstrated in the work of Souza and Candido (2010).

One of the main concepts of CBT is the identification of negative or distorted automatic thoughts that can contribute to pathological emotional states. This awareness allows the individual to question and challenge these thought patterns, replacing them with more balanced and realistic thoughts.

In addition to cognitive work, CBT incorporates behavioral interventions, strategies such as gradual exposure to feared situations, and problem-solving techniques that aim to modify maladaptive behaviors, promoting adaptation to challenging situations.

The effectiveness of CBT treatment has been demonstrated in a variety of anxiety and depression disorders and other psychiatric disorders as described by Butler, A. C. et al. (2006), due to its adaptability and practical focus make it valuable in different clinical contexts.

This form of treatment not only offers effective tools to deal with emotional and behavioral challenges but also enables individuals to become active agents in their change process, being a fundamental therapeutic intervention in promoting well-being. Mental being as described by Aaron Beck in his studies.

Treatment of Anxiety and Depressive Disorders—Pharmacological Treatment

Pharmacological treatment in psychiatry encompasses several drug classes with their respective psychotropic medications and their specific mechanism of action to treat different mental disorders.

The option to prescribe the medication will be based on the assessment of the signs and symptoms that the patient presents and based on diagnostic criteria, the health professional, usually a psychiatrist, will assess the need to prescribe medication on an individual basis to the patient.

Follow-up with regular consultations is necessary to evaluate possible side effects, dosage adjustments, and the possibility of combining medications to optimize results to improve the condition.

Pharmacological treatment for anxiety disorders aims to provide symptomatic relief for a better quality of life for patients. Several classes of medications are used, with choices based on the severity of symptoms, individual medical history, and treatment tolerance. Presented by Sadock and Sadock (2007), Selective Serotonin Reuptake Inhibitors (SSRIs), examples of which are sertraline and escitalopram, which act by increasing the levels of serotonin, a neurotransmitter associated with the regulation of anxiety. In addition, we have other drug classes such as Serotonin and Norepinephrine Reuptake Inhibitors (SNRIs), such as venlafaxine, desvenlafaxine, and duloxetine, and the tricyclic class, such as amitriptyline and clomipramine, which can be effective in treating disorders of anxiety. Benzodiazepines, such as diazepam, alprazolam, and clonazepam, provide quick relief from anxiety, but prolonged use can lead to dependence, and are generally prescribed in the short term and cases of acute anxiety attacks. There are also other classes of medications such as beta-blockers, such as propranolol that reduce the physical symptoms of anxiety, in addition to other classes that include buspirone and pregabalin which help control anxiety symptoms.

As already mentioned for the treatment of anxiety disorders, for depressive disorders, according to Sadock, we also use Selective Serotonin Reuptake Inhibitors (SSRIs), Selective Serotonin and Norepinephrine Reuptake Inhibitors (SSRIs), which are widely prescribed medications aimed at improving mood and reduce symptoms. In addition to these drug classes, we have other classes such as tricycles and Monoamine Oxidase Inhibitors (MAOS), among other drug classes, which are also options for treatment.

However, the choice of the medication class, as well as the medication, is based on the profile of each patient in a personalized way, considering the severity of symptoms, medical history, potential side effects, and socioeconomic conditions. Furthermore, regular follow-up with mental health professionals is essential to adjust medication as necessary and monitor possible adverse reactions and dose adjustments.

Cognitive-Behavioral Therapy for Anxiety Disorders

There are evidence that cognitive and behavioral therapies are effective for the treatment of anxiety disorders, with an impact on improving clinical conditions including panic disorder, generalized anxiety disorder, and social anxiety disorder, according to Cuijpers et al. (2016a, b). For patients with anxious symptoms, according to Beck (2013), an approach to the interrelationship between thoughts, emotions, and behaviors is necessary, which includes some of the processes that we will discuss below.

The therapeutic process of CBT in anxiety disorders requires the therapist to help the patient recognize and evaluate anxious or catastrophic thoughts, promoting critical understanding and, from this, promoting cognitive restructuring, that is, replacing negative thoughts with more positive thoughts. Balanced, this will reduce the anxiety associated with distorted interpretations.

The exposure technique is carried out gradually and helps the patient to confront situations or stimuli that generate anxiety, this can desensitize the factors that trigger anxiety. There are strategies to deal with anxiety with relaxation training, such as deep breathing and progressive muscle relaxation, which are taught to reduce the physiological activation associated with anxiety. Furthermore, it is necessary to identify avoidant behaviors that can reinforce anxiety and the therapist must work with the patient to gradually overcome these avoidances, techniques discussed by Otto and Deveney (2005).

These elements of cognitive behavioral therapy make up a therapeutic process that aims to develop coping strategies and the patient learns to develop adaptive strategies, being a form of treatment for anxiety disorders, including panic disorder, as demonstrated by Gisele et al. (2008). The active involvement of the patient, monitoring thoughts, and practicing learned skills are fundamental aspects for the success of this type of therapy. As described by Dugas et al. (2010), for generalized anxiety disorder, the application of CBT in a group is highly effective, in addition to individual therapy, and it has been proven that symptoms improve continuously throughout therapeutic follow-up and after treatment end of treatment.

Cognitive-Behavioral Therapy for Depressive Disorders

Treatment with Cognitive-Behavioral Therapy for depression aims to modify negative thought patterns and maladaptive behaviors associated with this disorder.

According to Beck et al. (2011), an initial assessment must be carried out by the therapist to understand depressive symptoms, identifying negative automatic thoughts and dysfunctional behavioral patterns to identify the most urgent and accessible problem.

Once the presence of negative behaviors and thoughts is identified, it is necessary to establish therapeutic goals to direct the treatment, providing a clear sense of direction for the patient. Throughout treatment, the patient must undergo cognitive restructuring, with the identification of negative automatic thoughts to replace these distorted thoughts with more balanced and realistic thoughts as described by Powell, V. B. et al. (2008).

A positive reinforcement schedule is necessary for the patient to engage in pleasurable activities, even if they initially seem challenging. This positive reinforcement is responsible for increasing motivation. This entire treatment process must be carried out through emotional self-regulation exercises: the patient learns to recognize, accept, and regulate negative emotions, developing strategies to face situations as described by Moorey (2010).

With the stability of the condition, the patient is exposed to activities to overcome the avoidance associated with depression and its symptoms. The therapeutic process must include the prevention of depressive relapses and strategies are developed to identify early signs of relapse, thus making preventive interventions possible.

As Beck describes, CBT is structured to promote practical tools to improve mood and general functionality, being one of the forms of treatment for depressive episodes with a focus on practical resolution of coping with daily challenges, contributing to a feeling of competence and control.

Pharmacological Treatment Associated with Cognitive-Behavioral Therapy for Anxiety and Depressive Disorders

Cognitive-behavioral therapy and drug treatment represent a way of managing anxiety and depressive disorders as individual treatments, but their combination increases the effectiveness of the treatment, as reported by Nakagawa, A. et al. (2017). Studies demonstrated by Wiles et al. (2014), indicate that resistant depression also presents a more adequate response to this association, as shown by the fact that this therapeutic integration reduces the financial costs dedicated to treatment. This combined therapy combines the role of CBT in changing thought and behavior patterns with the benefits of pharmacological intervention, aiming to provide patients with a more complete and personalized approach to recovery.

In the context of anxiety and depressive disorders, CBT helps patients recognize and challenge automatic negative thoughts, promoting their replacement with more realistic and constructive thoughts. This process contributes to changing behaviors associated with symptoms, promoting a gradual improvement in quality of life.

However, CBT may encounter limitations when symptoms are intense and active patient participation is challenging. In these cases, the introduction of drug treatment can play a fundamental role. Antidepressants and anxiolytics are frequently prescribed to stabilize the levels of brain neurotransmitters, providing symptom relief, and facilitating the effectiveness of cognitive-behavioral therapy, with this association being a faster response than monotherapy alone, described by Lopez and Basco (2015).

Collaboration between psychotherapists and psychiatrists is essential in the effective integration of these approaches, as discussed by Cooper, A. A. et al. (2016). Constant communication between healthcare professionals allows for appropriate adjustments in therapy and medication, considering the patient's response. Furthermore, it is essential to actively involve the patient in the decision-making process, clarifying expectations and promoting treatment adherence.

It is important to emphasize that the integrated approach does not mean a one-size-fits-all approach. Each individual is unique, and treatment must be adapted according to the patient's specific needs and characteristics. The combination of CBT and medication treatment not only alleviates immediate symptoms but also strengthens the patient's ability to deal with future challenges, contributing to a more sustainable recovery.

In summary, the integration of cognitive behavioral therapy with pharmacological treatment represents a comprehensive and personalized approach to anxiety and depressive disorders. Combining the benefits of cognitive and behavioral modification with neurobiological stabilization through medication, not only alleviates symptoms but also empowers patients to face emotional challenges more effectively.

Conclusion

In conclusion, the association between pharmacological treatment and cognitive-behavioral therapy represents an effective approach to coping with anxiety and depressive disorders due to the benefits of cognitive and behavioral modification offered by therapy and associated with the stabilization provided by medical treatments, a favorable scenario is created for the patient's full recovery.

This integrated approach not only aims for symptom remission but also promotes long-term emotional empowerment. By empowering patients with cognitive tools and coping strategies, along with pharmacological support, when necessary, the association between cognitive behavioral therapy and medication treatment provides a solid foundation for sustainable recovery and continuous quality improvement of life.

References

Beck, J. S. (2013). *Terapia cognitivo-comportamental: Teoria e prática*. Artmed.

Beck, A. T., & Alford, B. A. (2011). *Depressão: Causas e tratamento* (2nd ed.). Artmed.

Butler, A. C., Chapman, A. J., Formam, E. M., & Beck, A. T. (2006). The empirical status of cognitive-behavioral therapy: A review of meta-analyses. *Clinical Psychology Review, 26*(1), 17–31.

Cooper, A. A., et al. (2016). The therapeutic alliance and therapist adherence as predictors of dropout from cognitive therapy for depression when combined with antidepressant medication. *Journal of Behavior Therapy and Experimental Psychiatry, 50*, 113–119.

Cuijpers, P., Cristea, I. A., Karyotaki, E., Reijnders, M., & Huibers, M. J. H. (2016a). How effective are cognitive behavior therapies for major depression and anxiety disorders? A meta-analytic update of the evidence. *World Psychiatry, 15*, 245–258.

Cuijpers, P., Gentili, C., Banos, R. M., Garcia-Campayo, J., Botella, C., & Cristea, I. A. (2016b). Disorders relative effects of cognitive and behavioral therapies on generalized anxiety disorder, social anxiety disorder and panic disorder: A meta-analysis. *Journal of Anxiety Disorders, 43*, 79–89.

Dugas, M. J., Brillon, P., Savard, P., Turcotte, J., Gaudet, A., Ladouceur, R., Leblanc, R., & Gervais, N. J. (2010). A randomized clinical trial of cognitive-behavioral therapy and applied relaxation for adults with generalized anxiety disorder. *Behavior Therapy, 41*(1), 46–58.

Gisele, G. M., et al. (2008). Terapia cognitivo-comportamental no transtorno de pânico. *Revista Brasileira de Psiquiatria, 30*(Suppl 2). https://doi.org/10.1590/S1516-44462008000600005

Knapp, P., & Beck, A. T. (2008). Fundamentos, modelos conceituais, aplicações e pesquisa na terapia cognitiva. *Revista Brasileira de Psiquiatria, 30*(2), 54–64.

Lopez, M. A., & Basco, M. A. (2015). Effectiveness of cognitive behavioral therapy in public mental health: Comparison to treatment as usual for treatment resistant depression. *Administration and Policy in Mental Health, 42*(1), 87–98.

Moorey, S. (2010). The six cycles maintenance model: Growing a "vicious flower" for depression. *Behavioural and Cognitive Psychotherapy, 38*(2), 173–184.

Nakagawa, A., et al. (2017). Effectiveness of supplementary cognitive-behavioral therapy for pharmacotherapy-resistant depression: A randomized controlled trial. *Journal of Clinical Psychiatry, 78*(8), 1126–1140.

Otto, M. W., & Deveney, C. (2005). Cognitive-behavioral therapy and the treatment of panic disorder: Efficacy and strategies. *The Journal of Clinical Psychiatry, 66*(Suppl 4), 28–32.

Powell, V. B., Abreu, N., De Oliveira, I. R., & Sudak, D. (2008). Terapia cognitivo- comportamental da depressão. *Revista Brasileira de Psiquiatria, 30*(Suppl II), S73–S80.

Sadock, B. J., & Sadock, V. A. (2007). *Compêndio de psiquiatria. Ciência do Comportamento e Psiquiatria Clínica. Trad. de Claudia Dornelles et al* (9th ed.). Artmed.

Souza, I. C. W., & Candido, C. F. G. (2010). Diagnóstico psicológico e a terapia cognitiva: considerações atuais. *Revista Brasileira de Terapias Cognitivas, 5*(2), 82–92.

Wiles, N., et al. (2014). Clinical effectiveness and cost-effectiveness of cognitive behavioral therapy as an adjunct to pharmacotherapy for treatment-resistant depression in primary care: The CoBalT randomized controlled trial. *Health Technology Assessment, 18*(31), 1–137.

Index

A. C. Ornelas (ed.), *Transdiagnostic Approaches in Cognitive Behavioral Therapy*, https://doi.org/10.1007/978-3-031-63494-9

SPRINGER NATURE

GPSR Compliance

The European Union's (EU) General Product Safety Regulation (GPSR) is a set of rules that requires consumer products to be safe and our obligations to ensure this.

If you have any concerns about our products, you can contact us on ProductSafety@springernature.com

In case Publisher is established outside the EU, the EU authorized representative is:

Springer Nature Customer Service Center GmbH
Europaplatz 3
69115 Heidelberg, Germany

The manufacturer's authorised representative in the EU is Springer Nature Customer Service Centre GmbH, Europaplatz 3, 69115 Heidelberg, Germany. If you have any concerns regarding our products, please contact ProductSafety@springernature.com

Printed and bound by CPI Group (UK) Ltd, Croydon, CR0 4YY
01/10/2026
02225971-0002